THINGS YOU SHOULD KNOW ABOUT TEETH

The complete guide to Dental Health and Beauty

BENJAMIN LEE, B.D.S.

AuthorHouse™ UK Ltd.
500 Avebury Boulevard
Central Milton Keynes, MK9 2BE
www.authorhouse.co.uk
Phone: 08001974150

©2007 Benjamin Lee, B.D.S.. All rights reserved.

No part of this book may be reproduced, stored in a retrieval system, or transmitted by any means without the written permission of the author.

First published by AuthorHouse 9/17/2007

ISBN: 978-1-4343-1287-7 (sc)

Printed in the United States of America
Bloomington, Indiana

This book is printed on acid-free paper.

Dedication

To my parents William and Ivy for their love and always being there for me, and for teaching me to write composition from an early age. To my sister Rosalind and to my brother-in-law Timothy for their love and invaluable guidance during the making of this book. To my beautiful wife Hiroko, who has given me so much love, joy, dedication and kind support every single day and especially during life's many difficulties. To my uncle T.C.Foo for always being there to guide me whenever I am in need of help or advice. To my best friend Joerg Burmester who was, is and always will be my very best friend, and also to Kam who has always been ever so kind and supporting to me from the very first day we met.

To Peter Mayes, my kind housemaster and English tutor at boarding school who really taught me good English, and his wife Sue Mayes for her warmth and kindness during my 5 most memorable childhood years in Oxfordshire. To Adrienne Leon, my personal tutor who taught me all the dentistry I know, for her guidance, warmth and kindness which I will never forget.

Acknowledgements

I sincerely wish to thank Mr. Timothy Fitch and the talented staff at Authorhouse for their expertise in designing and putting all the material together in the making of this book. Their professionalism and enthusiasm sets new standards and their level of energy at work deserves great admiration. I also wish to thank Mr. Dean Shah for inspiring me to take the plunge and make this book.

Finally, and most importantly, I wish to thank Mr. Daniel Mok for all of his lovely artworks!

Preface.

Smiling is probably the most important and best facial expression for our social lives. We need to show teeth to make a really good smile. Smiles light up the face and always elicit smiles in return. In fact all facial expressions can be "better expressed" with the display of good teeth. Smiling enhances your attractiveness, glamour, popularity, confidence, self-esteem, sex-appeal, social life, and certainly success. There is an old Chinese saying that if you do not like to smile, you should never open a shop.

Celebrities heavily depend on their smiles. Facial expressions are able to reflect a person's state of mind, at all times, and it conveys this information to others who see you. When you smile to someone, it contains a whole lot of information about what's on your mind. A gleaming smile together with your friendly eyes shows people that you are delighted, and it says

"I like you very much and we can definitely get along just fine". It also implies your acceptance and approval of people, and it encourages them to approach you without the fear of rejection. Smiles are welcoming and they open doors. People who know they have great teeth have greater tendencies to smile readily. Friendly smiles also reflect the sincere and good nature of a person, and it radiates warm feelings in the atmosphere. It always looks nice, with thanks to the nice-looking teeth.

As the saying goes;

"If your face was never perfect, well at least your teeth can be; if your face is really perfect, then indeed your teeth must be. Smiling is an invaluable social tool for all the world to see; chewing is for eating well, a vital luxury."

Smiling is a good habit, it costs nothing and is easy to do. It always makes you look nice and at your very best. This alone can influence your success and your ultimate destiny. A winning smile with gleaming straight, white teeth looks glamorous, and it makes the best first impression. In the modern world, a good self-presentation and image is so important. Having good teeth is always an advantage.

This book gives you an understanding of how to first achieve the perfect smile starting with health, namely how to bypass all the common problems which cause harm to teeth. Preserving teeth intact throughout life is the main goal. Losing teeth is no longer an inevitable part of aging as once believed. It's either caused by infections, trauma, or bad dentalworks and these are all preventable. If you can be fully aware of all the ten main factors which threaten the integrity of your teeth, you will be in a much better position to safeguard against them. In any battle, you must know who and where all your enemies will attack you. Prevention is better than the cure and this principle applies especially to dental health. Human teeth lack the ability to regenerate, unlike other body tissues such as skin, hair, bone and nails, and henceforth all damages inflicted are permanent. If for instance, skin, hair, bone and nails failed to regenerate and were seriously damaged, they too would be difficult to repair or replace. How would you cope with losing all your fingernails, perhaps through fungal infections, and they never grew back? Teeth do require extra attention and care because they are constantly subjected to daily abuses, and the mouth is quite a hostile environment which threatens their existence.

Healthy teeth should already give you the perfect smile, but if you should endeavor to further enhance the beauty of your smile for your added attractiveness, there are various methods to do so and cosmetic dentistry has become very popular in recent years.

Everyone deserves to have good teeth, and it doesn't have to cost an arm or a leg. If they are well looked after from the very beginning, they are already pretty perfect. If there are problems with them, money is wisely spent to correct all of the past mistakes. From this point onwards, all you'll have to do is to maintain them "perfect as they are" all life long and never allow them to deteriorate. It's all a question of standards and these efforts cost next to nothing. Remember, losing teeth is the beginning of aging and silent suffering. If you really treasure your pearly whites like precious gems in your mouth then you will be on the right track to having good teeth for life.

Let this book guide you all the way.

Benjamin Lee, B.D.S.

Contents

Dedication	III
Acknowledgements	IV
Preface.	V
1. Anatomy	1
2. Why Are Teeth Important?	5
3. Prevention, Starting With Children	10
4. The Ten Key Causes Of "Toothaches And Tooth Losses"	18
5. Gum Disease	19
6. Overcrowding	24
7. Dental Cavities	30
8. Self-inflicted Wear	45
9. Wisdom Teeth	48
10. Infections	52
11. Smoking	54
12. Dental Trauma	55
13. Old Fillings And Overhangs	58
14. Missing Teeth	60
15. Cosmetic dentistry	69
16. Positioning Teeth	75
17. Whitening Teeth	79
18. Cosmetic Restorations	89
19. Gummy Smiles	91
20. Bad Breath-You Are Always The Last Person To Know	92
21. Food For Teeth	94
22. Things You Should Know About BRUSHING	97
23. Regular Care	104
24. Dental Phobia !	107
25. A List Of 20 Precautions.	111
Further Reading.	113
Index	115

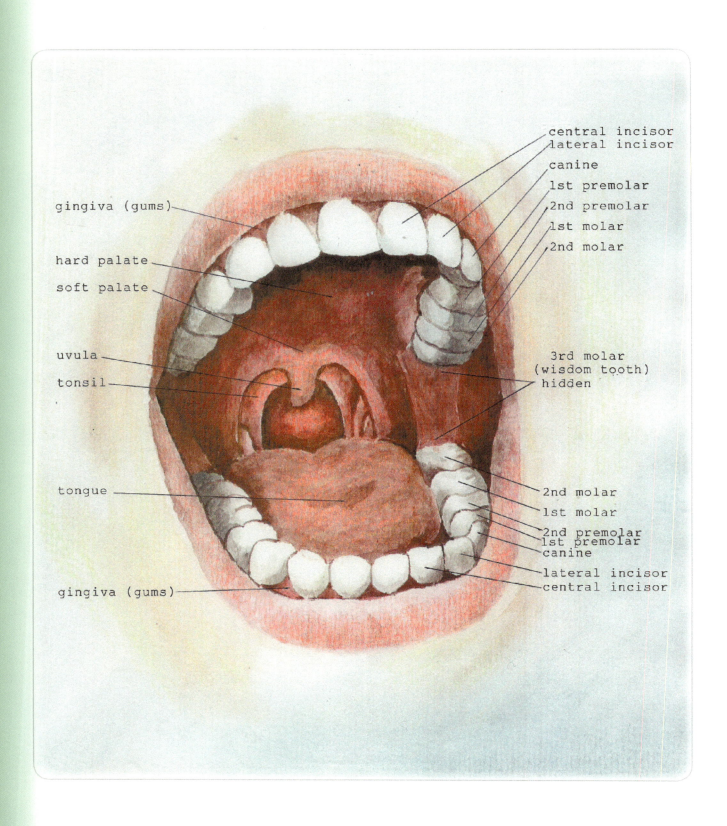

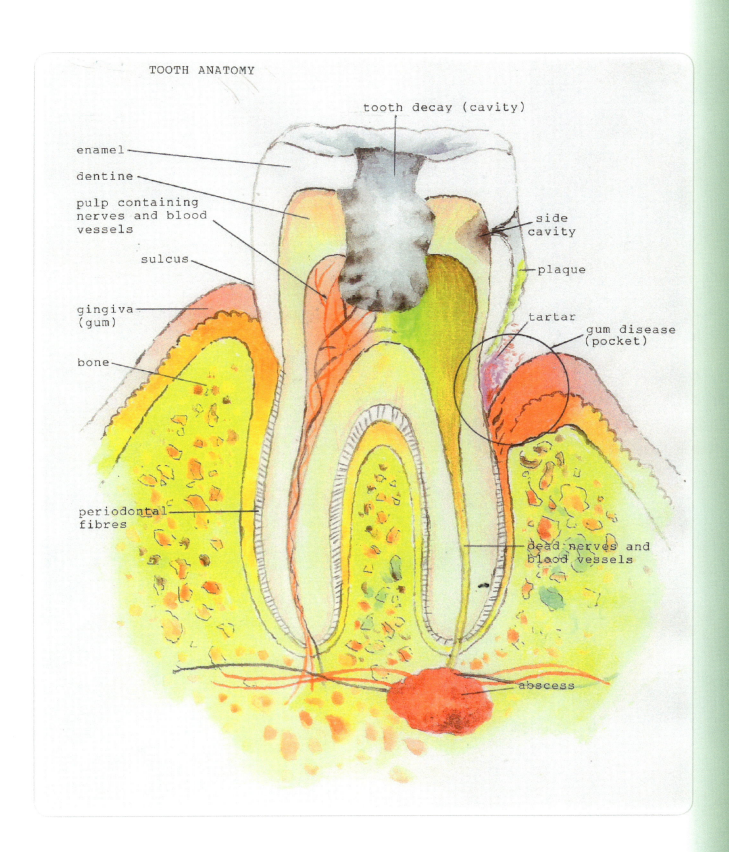

1. Anatomy

Before we begin, in order to understand what and where everything is in your mouth, it is helpful to have a basic understanding of the teeth and the basic oral anatomy.

The Oral Cavity

As the mouth opens, we enter into the oral cavity which serves many functions, and it is the first point of entry for the food to be introduced into our digestive organs. The oral cavity serves to provide a sensory analysis of the food material before it is swallowed. The teeth in the oral cavity mechanically processes the food, chopping them down to form a bolus when it is mixed with the saliva excreted from the salivary glands.

The skin lining of the oral cavity is known as the oral mucosa, and although nutrients are not absorbed in the oral cavity, the oral mucosa at the bottom of the tongue can be able to rapidly absorb some fat-soluble drugs, such as nitroglycerin which is placed under the tongue for the immediate relief of a heart attack. It travels to the heart to cause immediate dilatation of the blocked coronary artery there to resume the normal passage for blood-flow. This is a life-saving feature of the mouth ! Conversely the mouth can also be potentially harmful for your health as it houses an immense wealth of bacteria. The junction between the tooth and the gums (gingiva) at the gum line is known as the dentogingival (tooth-gum) junction. The gums cuff around each tooth to form a watertight seal. This dentogingival junction is the prime site for gum infections to occur and bacteria can leak into the bloodstream to infect the heart valves. Bacteria which accumulates there circumferentially around each tooth produces enzymes which are toxic and destroys the natural seal. If allowed to remain bacteria gains entry down the surface of the root to cause gum disease. Daily brushing at this "gum line" denies bacteria the chance to reside and to gain any initial entries into the gums.

Types Of Teeth. There Are Essentially 4 Different Types Of Teeth.

I: INCISORS –These are screwdriver shaped teeth, like chisels, with single roots at the front of the mouth used for cutting into food, as you may use it to bite into an apple, or cut spaghetti. They are the very front teeth we need most for smiling, in particular those upper two front teeth. There are 8 of these in both the child and adult dentition.

C: CANINES – These are conical shaped single rooted teeth with a pointed tip, at the 4 corners of the mouth, and are our longest teeth used to dig into food for shearing . They can also serve to guide the jaws during side to side excursions, rather like reference pillars. Canines are situated between the incisors and the premolars, and erupt later than them, often resulting in them erupting outside of the dental arch, due to the lack of space. The best way to describe them is by referring to them as the fangs of tiger teeth, or the prominent sharp Dracula teeth at the corners of their mouths. Without them our smile looks odd and they should always be retained even when they typically grow high up in the gums in a crowded dentition. People who never thought of wearing braces used to extract these "out-of-place" canines as a short cut solution. The smile looks narrow and "parrot-like" as a result and it also looses symmetry. There are 4 of these in both the child and adult dentition.

P: PREMOLAR-These have two cusps, and grind food. Premolar teeth do not exist in the child dentition, as there are no baby premolar teeth, but they are preceded by the baby molars. The baby molars occupy and reserve the spaces for them to eventually erupt into as they naturally shed at about the age of 10. There are 8 premolars in the adult dentition and they are commonly the teeth of first choice for extractions prior to wearing braces. Even if 4 premolar teeth were extracted to allow space for the rest of the teeth to straighten, there still remains 4 full-functioning premolars.

M: MOLARS –These teeth serve primarily for the major grinding of the food and they can exert heavy forces with their large flat surface areas. They have 4 cusps or more, and we use them for heavy duty food chewing and crushing. There are in total 12 molars in the adult dentition, but there is typically inadequate space for all of them in the mouth, and the 4 wisdom teeth, or the 3rd molars which erupt after adolescence are usually extracted, and most adults suffice with their 8 molars.

In particular the 1st molars are the first and most important adult molars to erupt into the mouth, at around the age of 6.

They are larger and occupy the best positions in the jaws for effective chewing, but are sadly commonly lost due to tooth decay subsequent to being heavily bathed in sugar from such early age. These are the very teeth which keep dentists busy either for their repeated repairs or their replacements. They are best protected by fissure sealants as soon as they erupt.

The Tooth

The tooth is a complex multilayered structure, containing nerve and blood supply within its core, supplying sensation.

It is divided into the crown, the neck, and the root. Enamel is white and covers most of the crown. It is the hardest natural structure in the body. The bulk of the underlying tooth consists mainly of dentine which is yellow, and as it houses nerve fibres, it is a very sensitive structure.

Any sensation felt is always of pain, and the tooth cannot distinguish hot from cold, or other variations of stimuli.

The neck of the tooth, at the gum line, marks the boundary between the crown of the tooth, which projects into the oral cavity, and the root which is embedded within the bone. The central bulk of the tooth consists mainly of dentine, a mineralized matrix similar to that of bone, but at the very centre of this structure situates the central nerve and blood vessel complex in the form of the dental pulp, which enters it right at the tip, or apex, of the root via a small hole known as the apical foreman, providing sensation and nutrients to the tooth.

The space which houses these vital tissues within the crown of the tooth is known as the pulp cavity, and that space within the root is known as the root canal. Extensions of nerve fibres penetrate a third or more of the way across into the dentine structure, accounting for the sensitivity of dentine when it is directly exposed to the mouth.

Dentine structure is yellower and softer than enamel, and it is possible to be worn away (commonly by heavy toothbrushing).

Enamel is the hardest material of the body and it contains calcium phosphate in a crystalline form, or calcium hydroxyapatite. However, it is brittle in nature, and will readily crack on an impact to it. It is also very white in colour, and whitest when it is of a new tooth, when in full thickness. It is the most superficial protective layer of the tooth and is formed overlying the dentine at the crown. However with wear and tear throughout life, enamel becomes thinner and the yellowness of dentine becomes more apparent. As a result people tend to show more yellow teeth as they age. Chewing, grinding, toothbrushing, and recurrent exposure of acidic foods (citrus fruits, acidic drinks), can all collectively contribute to the imminent wear of enamel.

Enamel connects to dentine at their interface, known as the Enamel-Dentine Junction, or EDJ, and this is a plane of weakness. In certain conditions where there is imperfect formation of either the enamel structure (Amelogenesis Imperfecta) or dentine structure (Dentinogenesis Imperfecta), the enamel will readily shear away at this junction. Another example is when there is tooth decay, the decay penetrates through the tiny hole created in the enamel, the bacteria will spread sideways across this plane of weakness to dissolve a larger area of dentine, to proceed directly downwards toward the dental pulp. When all of the dentine underneath is softened by decay, the shell of enamel will suddenly crumble. Tooth decay affects dentine faster and more extensively than enamel once it is reached, resulting in a cavity. At the root of the tooth, the dentine is surrounded by a similar hard structural layer known as cementum, which is connected by collagen fibres, the periodontal ligament fibres, to the bone surface. These fibres are able to provide some degree of movement of the tooth itself during chewing, acting as shock-absorbers. They have nerves to provide a most efficient proprioceptive mechanism for tactile sensations; as for example, when there is a wafer-thin piece of paper between your teeth, you can sense it.

The Gums

The gums are also known as the gingiva, and cuffs around the teeth at the neck, to form the gingival margin, or gum line.

There is also some attachment to the tooth itself, just below the gum line, within which lies a gutter of space known as the gingival sulcus approximately 2mm in depth around the neck of the tooth and commonly collects dental plaque. This pocket of space is the starting area for gum disease and tooth brushing to remove bacteria from here is absolutely mandatory.

2. Why Are Teeth Important?

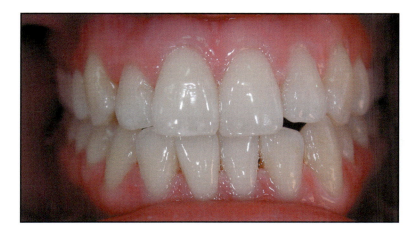

Having good teeth is all about the quality of life and as we advance in age, the ability to eat well becomes fundamentally important. A beautiful radiant smile that does show healthy and natural teeth is one of the greatest assets any person can ever have and the mouth is always a focus of attention. Teeth can have a profound influence on face appearances, and the smile can leave a best first impression on others before a word is uttered. Once you have a smile which displays great looking teeth it could be the greatest and most essential social tool any person can have. It brings joy to others and the gesture of smile always elicits smiles in return. In today's culture we are often judged by our outward appearances and a neat and a tidy-looking set of natural teeth displayed on the face serves not only to express the meticulous nature of a person, but it also indicates a person's affluence and good socio-economic status. Glamour starts with good personal hygiene and healthy teeth do symbolize health, youth and vitality. No costs are spared in the relentless pursuit of health and an immaculate image.

Our teeth serve so many purposes in our daily lives that we would be in dire straits without them. The enjoyment of food is one of life's greatest luxuries. Most of us could never imagine losing them during our lifetimes because we were born with them and so, what could go wrong?! Our teeth gives us strength and confidence, and the jaws which cannot clench comfortably on a complete and solid set of teeth is intolerable. This undermines the function of the mouth and gives rise to all sorts of jaw clickings and discomforts. We need to take for granted that the whole teeth that we already have would never be confiscated by disease, but sadly people still do lose them today as a result of unnecessary damages. The average person, even in advanced countries, can lose up to 10 teeth by the age of 50 and up to a third of people over the age of 75 today have lost all their teeth. Millions of dollars are spent every year for repairing and replacing teeth, but in fact, human teeth were structurally built to last for a lifetime. Enamel is after all the hardest structure in the human body. The psychological effects of losing teeth can be devastating. Some people who have lost many teeth begin to retreat into themselves, avoid many social activities they would have otherwise enjoyed, and hesitate to meet new friends they could otherwise have developed close relationships. They can lose confidence and self-esteem. Children and young people with bad-looking teeth can also suffer the same adverse effects; if they are very crooked or are grossly discoloured.

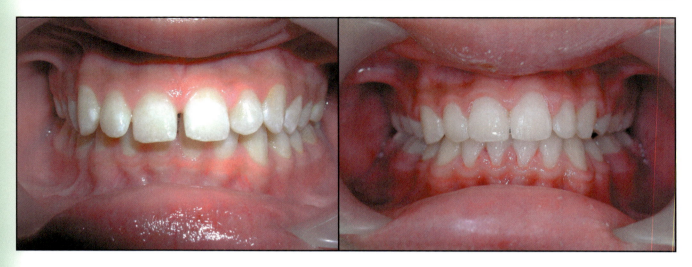

The effects on any person having their smile restored are most dramatic, almost like bringing them back to life! They smile more, talk more, sing more, dominate parties with their cheerful smiles, and are generally more sociable afterwards. The correction of a smile is one of the most appreciated and gratifying services a dentist can render to a patient and the repairs of tooth damages, replacement of missing teeth, and the orthodontic straightening of crooked teeth for children, teenagers and adults forms an important part of the profession. However, the primary aim in the field of dentistry is to prevent all oral diseases.

Smiling, Talking, Singing, Laughing.

Whenever you smile for a photo, you tend to smile at your very best because photographic images will last forever. Most people could not even step out of their homes without their two front teeth, if for example, the post-crowns had dropped out! In the past, women had their ugly rotten and crooked teeth extracted to make false teeth before their weddings, just for the sake of smiling.

It was a simple solution for them because wearing braces and having white fillings were afforded only by the wealthy.

Life is never the same with many teeth lost and a set of false teeth always tend to feel uncomfortable and unnatural. Plastic alternatives in false teeth compromises talking, singing and chewing and they could never match natural good teeth. Front teeth are very important for pronouncing words and sounds and the clarity of speaking coming from the natural teeth could never be superseded by any false replicas. It is fair to say that all human tissues replaced artificially are never quite as good, yet costly. Teeth are vital for pronouncing "T", "CH", "F" and "S" sounds. The upper front teeth are very important.

For example; Try to say "FANCY" or any words starting with "F", without your lower lip touching your upper teeth.

Or try "I FANCY FAMOUS FRIENDS AND FIND THEM FABULOUS, FANTASTIC, FUN AND FULFILLS MY JOY".

Guiding Your Jaws.

Your mouth only functions if your jaws could move, and only the lower one does. The jaws need to close together on the teeth, and the comfortable way in which the jaws can close is determined by the way in which the teeth can bite. Good biting is very important, which is why wearing braces is such an essential part of growing up. The corrected changes are lifelong.

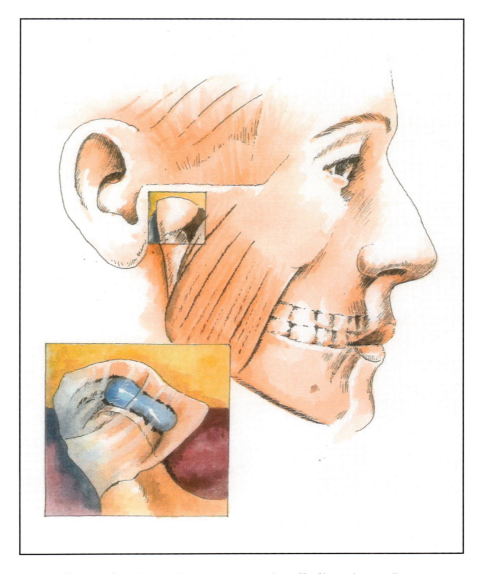

The jawjoints allows the lower jaw to move in all directions. Incorrect and imbalanced biting or chewing with too many teeth missing would cause it to feel pain. The jawjoint is also called the **TMJ** or the Temporomandibular Joint.

CHEWING

Good teeth determines our ability to eat all kinds of our favourite foods. Chewing is the first and most important stage of the digestion process when food is cut and ground by our teeth. This mincing increases the surface area of the foods to be exposed and mixed with the digestive enzymes from our saliva in order to break them down. Chewing makes the food softer and warmer, forming a bolus which can be readily swallowed and passed into the stomach for the next stage of digestion. The front teeth serve to cut the food first, but it is those back teeth which do most of the chewing. The consequences of tooth loss includes inadequate chewing which would lead to indigestion. People with less teeth in the mouth need to restrict themselves to a much softer diet, compromising their level of nutrition and their enjoyment of food.

FOR SUPPORTING THE FACE.

Teeth are important to maintain the shape of the face. They act like a fence barrier to prevent the collapse of the cheeks and the lips into the mouth. The front teeth can determine the profile of the lips. Teeth can also reduce the overall height of the face if they have been considerably shortened over time due to wear. People who grind their teeth will wear them down quicker.

People who have lost all their back teeth will also wear the remaining front ones quicker. As a result, the jaws close on shorter teeth, and the distance from the base of the nose to the bottom of the chin will be reduced. It is possible to restore the original heights of teeth with the provision of crowns (or caps) and will simultaneously restore the original height of the face, reversing also any wrinkles which resulted from the loss of face-height. Without teeth, there will be more wrinkles all around the lips.

PRESERVING THE JAWBONES.

If all the teeth roots are missing for too long, the jawbones will shrink. Wrinkles can appear on the face as a result of the diminutive jaws which form its underlying frame. Preserving natural teeth in the jaws, preserves the jaw skeleton which in turn preserves the overall original shape, form and height of the face; this in turn preserves one's youthful face-look.

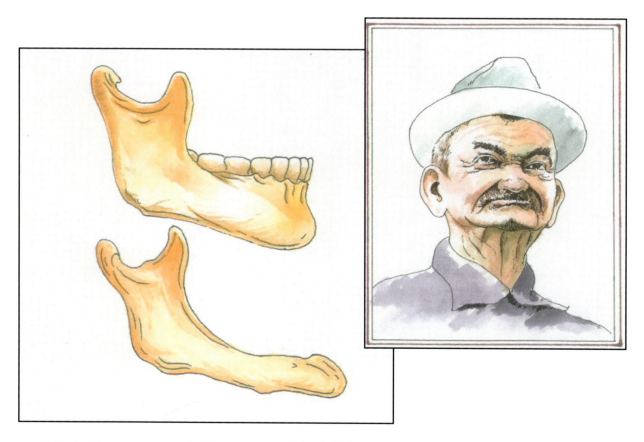

The jawbones can only be preserved in full form if there are healthy, natural tooth-roots embedded within them.

"TEETH ARE VERY IMPORTANT FOR ALL THE FUNCTIONS OF THE MOUTH".

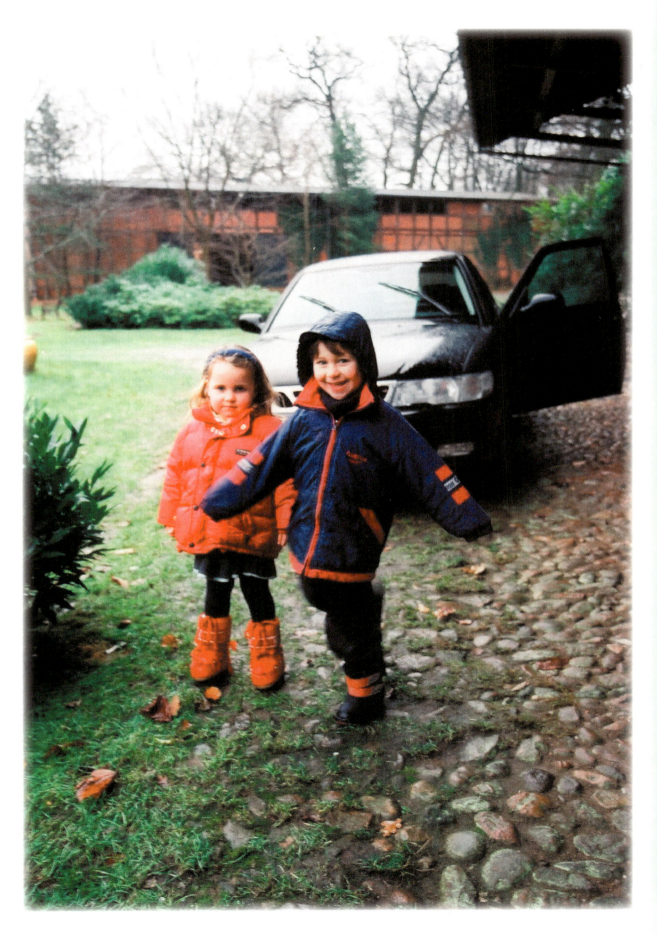

3. Prevention, Starting With Children

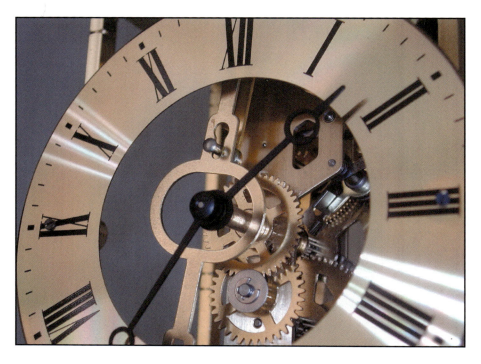

When to START ?!

It is ideal to start your child with your dentist as soon as there are teeth in the mouth, but this is often impractical. Brushing the teeth really should begin as soon as the front teeth are visible, as early as 6 months old. By the age of 2 and a half to 3 years old the child will have almost all of their 20 baby teeth when they are also probably more capable to understand things and are aware of their surroundings. This is perhaps a good time to take your child to your dentist.

Child dental clinics often consist of very comforting environments for your child as they have all the soft toys and children's books, sometimes even your child's favourite cartoons are showing in the little corner "baby's room".

The whole objective is to introduce dental surroundings to your child, especially the dental chair, and getting used to opening the mouth for inspections. Acceptance is always best when all procedures are fun, easy and painless and an event to look forward to. Initial anxieties are always inevitable, and it might be a good idea to begin with placing your child on your lap for the first few appointments, with you in the chair. You can open your mouth together with your child's.

This will become a series of training sessions, and most probably the first few visits will be focused on toothbrushing .

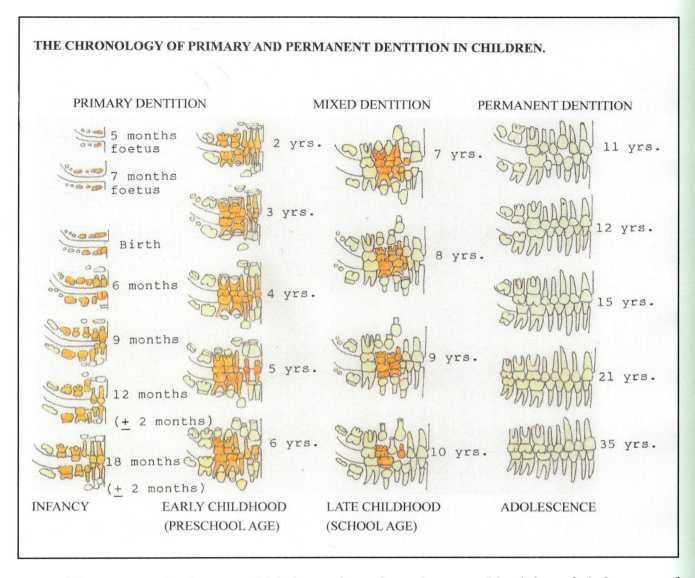

The reason why there are 20 baby teeth, and yet there are 32 adult teeth is because of the 8 adult premolars and the 4 wisdom teeth in the adult dentition. The 8 baby molar teeth are succeeded by 8 adult premolars whilst the adult molars develop behind.

This is only a general guide for tooth eruption timing and sequence. Some people have their teeth erupting earlier than others and a delay of up to 18 months for permanent teeth is considered normal and acceptable. In general the lower teeth erupt sooner than their opposing upper teeth, and the pattern always begins with the front teeth. However, the commonest reason for teeth not to erupt at all is either because they are naturally missing, as in wisdom teeth, the upper lateral incisors, or the lower second premolars; or that they are trapped underneath, as in the case of premolars caused by the early loss of baby molars, allowing the adult first molar to drift too far forwards; the wisdom teeth and canines, simply because there is no space for them.

Teething

This concerns most parents, as from the age of six months and until the age of 3. Children will start to erupt their baby teeth, usually starting with the lower front teeth. In most cases, there is no discomfort, but occasionally, there is some distress when there is irritation in the area of the gum above and around the erupting baby tooth, the gum being slightly swollen and red at times. It is often mildly irritating only, but is more discomforting for the larger baby molars when they begin to come out. Sometimes there may be red patches on the cheeks, slight fever, general irritability, crying, loss of appetite, sleeplessness dribbling of saliva, frequent loose stools, but these are mostly all related to the teething. If they are not eating, give them plenty of water to remain hydrated. A soft diet is useful but its only for one or two days. When the tooth finally erupts all normality returns, including the appetite.

There are all sorts of teething toys; teething rings, rattles and keys designed for the natural tendency to bite and suck to relieve the soreness with the pressure of biting on such devices, and they often work. There are also teething biscuits which are hard for their biting on and these relieve the child of the soreness. It is important that they contain no sugar or else tooth decay may result from this habit, or the child may develop a sweet tooth. Ointments and jellies are also available for application to the sore gums, and they also provide some pain relief. Sometimes a paracetamol child-dosage tablet provided by your doctor will give relief. Once the tooth erupts further, all the soreness, swellings, and all other associated problems will subside.

BRUSHING TEETH

As soon as a baby tooth erupts, even if it is the only one in the mouth, it must be brushed twice daily. There are all sorts of baby toothbrushes and fluoride toothpastes with all types of colours and flavours to choose from for young ages. Only the tiniest amount of toothpaste is really necessary, as they tend to swallow some anyway. Swallowing too much of the fluoride is not so good for your child as this may cause them to vomit. Brushing teeth must be an integral part of your child's routine care, train them to develop it as a routine daily habit. However the manual dexterity of children limits the effectiveness of their own brushing and parents must assist children in their brushing until they reach about the age of 6. Flossing is not necessary at these ages.

BOTTLE FEEDING (BABY BOTTLE CARIES)

Your child must never suck on a bottle for too long, as drinks usually contain some sugar. This could cause widespread dental decay to all surfaces of every tooth, known as rampant decay. If this happens, the whole mouth of baby teeth will all decay indiscriminantly front, sides and back, from molars to incisors. It is very destructive and hard to treat.

The most damage is done during sleeping, when the salivary flow is reduced. Night exposure to the sugar during sleep causes by far the most decay in the mouth and is usually caused by taking sugary snacks just before bedtime. For this reason, all teeth should be brushed and rinsed with water before bedtime, removing all the sugar beforehand. During the daytime, keep sweets away from your child as much as possible between mealtimes, and limit these to breakfast, lunch and dinner times only!

For the rest of the time, the saliva neutralizes all acids as it acts as a natural buffer. It is best also to avoid baby foods which contain sugar, and buy medicines which are sugar-free.

The Smile Of Children.

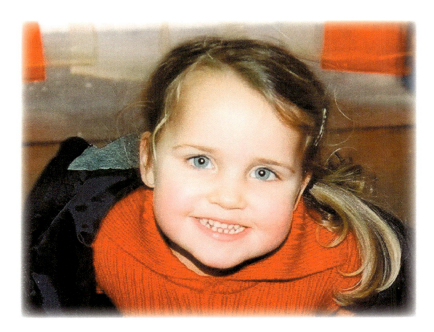

The sweetest smile of a young child always brings joy. Generally the smile of the baby teeth should show spaces between them. As baby teeth are considerably smaller than the adult teeth which follow, it is logical that there are spaces in-between.

If not, then it seems possible that all the adult teeth which eventually replace them will have to battle it amongst themselves for the limited space in the small jaw. It is not certain that the adult teeth will eventually be very crooked, as the jaws are still growing. This is hard to predict and perhaps they might grow large enough to accommodate them all in the end. Baby teeth which shows crowding or lack spaces between them is merely an early sign of things to come, but it is not as yet, for certain.

Dentists normally prefer to see spacing between baby teeth.

Thumbsucking.

Thumbsucking is very common for children but they usually cease the habit by around the age of 5. There is typically a hole at the front teeth for the thumb if the habit continues, which fits exactly, and they cannot come together as the back teeth bite together. This is known as an anterior open bite. There is also an increase in overjet at the front teeth. However all such unnatural positionings of teeth to form this front hole caused by this habit are completely self-correcting when the habit finally ceases and the teeth are repositioned back to their normal places under the influences of the lips and the tongue.

The First Visit.

It is actually difficult to answer when your child should first be brought to a dental visit. Ideally it should be as soon as the first tooth erupts, but the fact of the matter is that your child is perhaps too young to understand anything right after birth. However, it is best to introduce children to dentists when they do begin to understand things. A first visit is often just an introduction to the environment and to familiarize the child with the dental chair, the warm friendly dentist, and to learn how to brush. Children's books on dental topics and fun things to play with at the dental office will make the child feel comfortable, and even look forward to regular visits. They must never be allowed to suffer any discomforting treatments. Dental prevention must be exercised to the fullest, not only because children are very susceptible to getting decay and toothaches, but more because they are not likely to tolerate any injections in the mouth, face the drill, or face up to an extraction !!The whole objective with dental prevention is to protect your child from ever needing a single filling, and it's possible.

THE WORST SITUATION.

The worst case scenario is the "First Visit Emergency Experience", when the child has a severe toothache and had never seen a dentist before. The sight of a huge needle forced into his mouth will always be conceived to be painful and it will be remembered for a very long time. The aftermath of this type of event will be likely to be lifelong lingering in his mind.

The word "terror" doesn't even describe it and he will likely suffer from "Dental Phobia" onwards throughout life. Sometimes a very anxious child with too many cavities may need to have all the treatments done "one-time" under a general anaesthesia in a dental hospital.

BABY MOLARS

Baby teeth easily fall victim to tooth decay and are commonly extracted as a result. Baby molar teeth, however, should always be restored and retained until they shed naturally because they serve to guide the eruption of adult premolars into their correct positions. If not, the early extraction of baby molar teeth can have devastating consequences. They can no longer serve to hold back the adult 1st molar tooth existing behind them from the age of 6, and it will tip forwards to block the space intended for the premolars. The premolars do succeed the baby molar teeth but are still developing and are not due to erupt until the age of 10.

Baby molars do not contain deep enough fissures to warrant fissure sealants, hence topical fluoride and good brushing suffices.

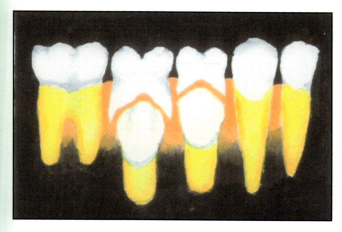 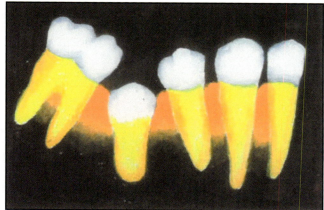

A　　　　　　　　　　　　　　　　　　　B

Fig. A : The baby molar teeth occupy the spaces needed for the normal eruption of the premolars.

Fig. B : If the baby molar teeth are destroyed by tooth decay and are extracted early, the large 1st adult molar will tip forwards into the space trapping the premolars. This is a difficult situation to reverse and it must be avoided at all costs.

Stainless Steel Crowns

Every effort is made to restore even the badly decayed baby molar. In such events, they may need to be crowned and crowns made of stainless steel are cheap and practical. This will maintain the tooth for chewing functions. It is always best to preserve baby molar teeth until their natural shedding at about the age of 10.

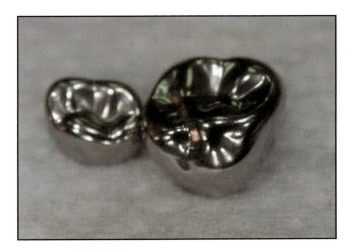
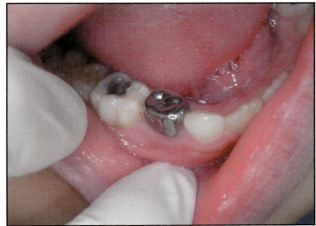

Space Maintainers

Space maintainers are provided in the event that a baby molar tooth has to be extracted early.

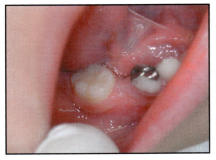
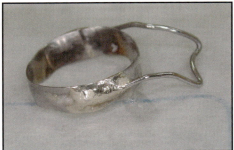
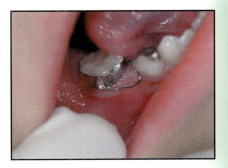

Prevention Steps.

1. Fluoride Treatments

Fluoride is by far the most important mineral for teeth and incorporating it into the structure is a first major step forwards.

Fluoride gel topically applied to teeth incorporates fluoride mineral into the enamel structure. This forms a stronger surface layer with denser mineral to shield the tooth from decay. If the local water supply already contains fluoride, this treatment may be optional. However, if there is no fluoride in the water supply, this treatment should begin around the age of 3 and is repeated once or twice a year at the clinic. Always use a toothpaste which contains fluoride. With the abundance of sweets consumed by children nowadays the addition of fluoride minerals onto their teeth has become necessary for their protection.

2. **FISSURE SEALANTS**
The four first adult molars begin to erupt from about the age of 6 and they are positioned just behind the baby molars.

Fissure sealants should be applied to their deep fissures as soon as possible because they are highly prone to decay .

3. **ORTHODONTIC TREATMENT**
Between the ages of 7-13 children are shedding their baby teeth and the adult teeth erupt to replace them. This is known as the mixed dentition stage, during which time both the baby and adult teeth exist in the mouth. During this time, the gum line can allow bacteria to leak in and accumulate underneath the loosening baby tooth to cause gum abscesses. Children do have poorer manual dexterity and their imperfect brushing can result in more occurrences of gum abscesses and bleedings.

Regular twice-annual check-ups are imperative for them . They can also have their teeth polished and receive fluoride treatments. Any irregularities with tooth sheddings are dealt with quickly and the normal development of their adult teeth are monitored. If the adult teeth are growing into wrong positions, as in crossbites and severely protruding upper front teeth, orthodontic treatments using removable braces are done to correct them. The growth of their jaws are also monitored.

If one jaw is discovered to be growing longer than the other jaw, devices can be provided and worn full-time to control it.

At around the ages of 11-13 years, full orthodontic treatment must be considered and this need must be carefully assessed.

The need for orthodontic treatment is decided only after a thorough examination. If your child has a small mouth and the teeth are very crowded, the many stagnation areas between crowded teeth make it difficult for them to clean. Straightened teeth not only enables teeth to the kept clean better throughout life, but the correction of the bite is very important for the comfort of the jawjoints and jaw muscles. The chewing is more efficient, the smile is more attractive, and good oral hygiene is easier maintained when teeth are straight. Orthodontics sets the teeth up for a lifetime of good oral health. Adults are also well-advised to have their crooked teeth straightened for the same reason and it is never too late to start.

4. **WISDOM TEETH**
Wisdom teeth should be checked after the age of 17 to determine if they exist or are likely to cause problems in the future.

The best time to remove them is as soon as their crowns have erupted into the mouth whilst their roots are still short and have not fully grown. If they are growing at an angle they are likely to become impacted. Hesitations and delays to remove them, if already advised to do so, allows time for their roots to develop fully, and there's no telling that they may grow too crooked, bent, or form hooks at their tips . When they finally begin to cause unbearable infection problems they might become virtually impossible to remove. If the root-tips should embrace vital structures, such as a major nerve of the jaw, it would be very risky. Those wisdom teeth which are likely to cause problems in the future are best removed earlier. Impacted wisdom teeth not only can cause horrendous infections, but they can also cause the tooth in front of them to rot so badly that they too are extracted. Most people today do not have large enough jaws to accommodate all of their genetically programmed "32 adult teeth" because the modern soft diets require less chewing and the jaws no longer need to grow to their full potentials to support the muscles. As a result, the wisdom teeth being the last to erupt, are often trapped.

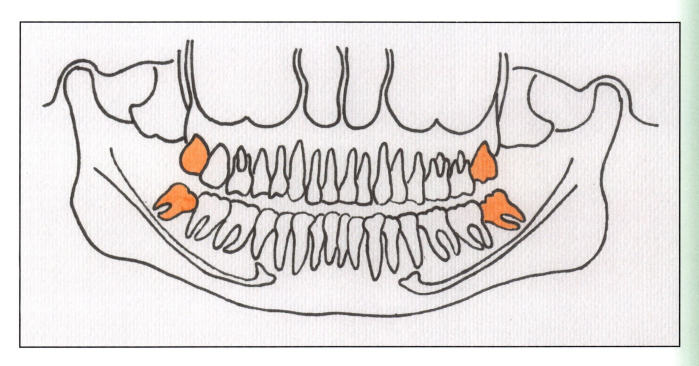

A PANORAMIC X-RAY WILL REVEAL THE WISDOM TEETH.

4. The Ten Key Causes Of "Toothaches And Tooth Losses"

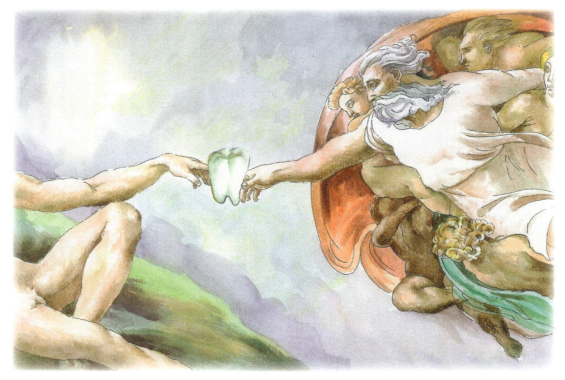

"Human teeth can never be replaced by man as good as they were given by nature".

There Are 10 Key Causes Of "Toothaches And Tooth Losses":

> Gum disease
> Overcrowding
> Dental cavities
> Self-inflicted wear
> Wisdom teeth
> Infections
> Smoking
> Dental trauma
> Old fillings and overhangs
> Missing teeth

In order to understand how to protect our teeth from being damaged, we must be completely aware of the ten major ways in which this can happen, as far as "the eye can see".
In dentistry, these could be conveniently remembered as the Ten Commandments for Toothaches and Tooth Losses if they are encoded in G-O-D-S-W-I-S-D-O-M. Let's go through them one by one to understand how they can lead to tooth damages, how they can be prevented and treated.

"People are often destroyed through a lack of knowledge".

5. Gum Disease

1. A mostly painless and slow disease caused by oral bacteria.
2. Causes adult teeth to become loosen and fall out.
3. Causes abscesses and spreads infection.
4. Prevented by good oral hygiene and regular scaling.
5. Major cause for tooth-loss.
6. There is no effective cure.
7. Influenced by nutrition, general health and immune system.
8. Accelerated by smoking.
9. Bacteria in the gums threatens the health of the heart. (Heart valves and coronary artery).

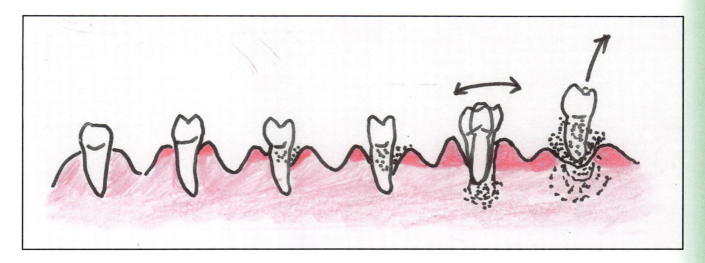

The Facts About Gum Disease.

Gum disease, (known as Periodontal Disease), painlessly damages the supporting structures around the tooth, (known as the Periodontium), causing the teeth to loosen and shed. This affects mainly adults and it is a major cause for tooth loss.

Oral bacteria, in the form of dental plaque, slips down our gum lines and causes the gums to peel away from the tooth. It does this by releasing toxins which destroys everything around it (rather like a solvent). It wipes out the gums, the collagen fibres attaching the tooth, and the bone around it. When the gums are peeled, the bone around it disappears and the tooth sheds.

There is never any serious pain from start to finish, and until the tooth finally sheds on your pillow, you'd never suspect it.

According to the latest UK Adult Dental Health Survey data 40%-45% of adults have moderate destructive gum disease, and 5-10% of adults have it in the advanced stages. It can affect young adults in their early 20's, but those who do have it almost always have very poor oral hygiene.

First Signs
1. The gums bleed every time you brush and floss.
2. The gums feel uncomfortable between the teeth.
3. Some of the teeth feel somewhat wobbly.
4. Biting is uncomfortable, and there feels a swelling in the gums at the back.
5. The gums can peel away from the teeth easily, revealing a lot of tartar inside.

What Causes It ?
It is now certain that gum disease is directly linked to the presence of bacteria in our mouths and plaque is the culprit.

With its presence, the rate and extent of the disease progression can also be influenced by our general health, immune system status, pregnancy, hormonal and nutritional status (Vitamin C), which makes some people more susceptible to it than others.

Smoking.
Smoking has harmful effects on the gums as it causes more tartar to form on the teeth. This is because the calcium concentration in the dental plaque of smokers is also remarkably higher than in non-smokers. The gums are also never as healthy in the presence of tobacco because it restricts the blood supply to the gums, giving them less nourishment.

Oral health generally deteriorates as a result.

Gingivitis is the inflammation of the gums which appears red, swollen, and are ready to bleed but it is usually not painful.

Children and adults alike can get gingivitis if they leave the bacteria sitting on their gums, but it is completely reversed with good toothbrushing and flossing.

Periodontitis is the inflammation of the "Periodontium" or the supporting structures around the root when bacteria had gone deeper under the gum line. As this happens, the gums peel away painlessly from the tooth to form a loose gum-cuff creating a pocket. The bacteria collects deep within it and as they can no longer be reached by the toothbrush they invade deeper. The bacteria, dead gum cells, blood, and toxins can form a soup of pus during the process which can either be trapped to form painful abscesses or it can leak painlessly out of the gum line. When it leaks out, it releases foul odours to give a bad breath, and whenever the tooth is sucked, it tastes salty. The pus could be passed from person to person with social contacts, as in kissing, sharing food or drinks (passing the bottle) at a party gathering. The gum infection can spread sideways to infect other teeth around it leading to their early losses.

Periodontitis is classified into Early, Moderate and Advanced stages depending on the extent of the damage, and it mainly affects adults, but in fact, most adults.

Gum Disease

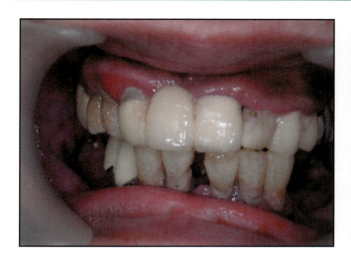
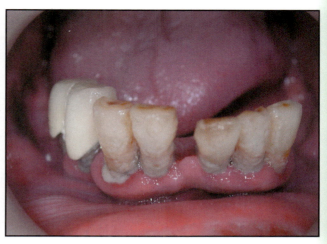

Advanced Periodontitis *"This Is Never Actually Painful, Believe It Or Not!"*

Prevention Measures.

1. Keeping a good oral hygiene is the main key to prevention. Brushing at the gum lines is particularly important to deny plaque their chance to enter into your gums at the fronts and backs of teeth. Flossing teeth is also important because it removes the plaque from between your teeth where they could otherwise accumulate and proceed with entry. Use of interdental brushes is most important if you have to clean under any dental bridges that you have in the mouth. If your toothbrush looks worn, and the bristles have all flared, you must change for a new one. Never use the same toothbrush for over 3 months.

    As it is virtually impossible to remove every single speck of plaque in the mouth, some will remain to form tartar.

2. Regular check-ups at least once a year is important to have your gum pockets checked. A regular scale & polish done once or twice a year is important and as there is no known cure available for gum disease, prevention in this way is the best and only form of treatment.

Treatments.

1. Scale & Polish

As tartar and stains will develop on your teeth regardless of your meticulous efforts, they must be removed professionally.

Professional cleaning removes all the bacteria, stains, tartar, and so on from your teeth, giving your gums a fresh start.

Hand scalers or ultrasonic machine scalers are used to gently scrape off the tartar and other tooth deposits above and just below the gum line. The polishing of the teeth removes plaque, stains and all else with rotating rubber cups and polishing pastes. No injections are needed for a scale and polish. All rough fillings are also polished, or replaced if necessary.

2. Deep Scaling.

If the roots are contaminated deeper by tartar and bacteria, these must be completely scraped clean with special instruments.

Under local anaesthesia, the infected tooth root is "root-planed" with sharp instruments, removing all tartar, stains, plaque, bacteria, toxins and pus. There is no method yet to induce the complete reattachment of loose gums back onto the tooth and regeneration of bone back to their former heights is, as yet, totally impossible. Once gum disease had passed beyond a certain point, the damage done is permanent. Deep scaling only helps to stabilize the problem.

3. Gum Surgery.

In the more severe forms when the disease had progressed too far down the roots, it is better to gain direct and open access to clean the infected roots with surgery. The loose gums are lifted away from the roots of teeth to allow a more thorough cleaning, and they are stitched back afterwards. This may seem like a more drastic approach but it is very necessary to be able to get right to the "root of the problem" and completely clean everything underneath.

4. Gingivectomy.

Another approach to the problem is by eliminating the pocket completely by cutting away the free-flapping gum tissues no longer attached to the roots. This has advantages and disadvantages. The main advantage is to be able to clear away the floppy gums sheltering bacteria, and allows the root surfaces to be openly exposed for daily brushing. This is known as a gingivectomy and is good for the long term survival of the tooth. It is often well-advised by the dentist. However, the disadvantage of removing the loose gums is that it reveals the problem in a smile. The exposed roots with gums absent around them appears unsightly and are also left uninsulated and can become very sensitive to hot and cold foods.

Gum disease causes extensive gum destruction which is so ghastly disfiguring that one could be deterred from smiling.

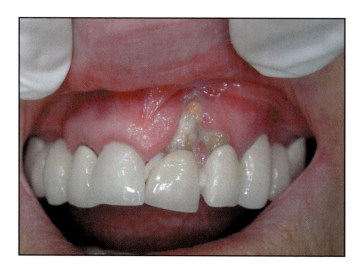

Gum Disease Is Real And Is Seriously Something
You Simply Cannot Smile About !

Teeth without gums or gum fleshes between them, showing unimaginable hollow gaps between their roots, cannot be satisfactorily restored by dental cosmetics. Please beware! Pink and firm gums which look healthy and scallop neatly around the necks of teeth is as vital to the smile as the conditions of the teeth themselves. A straight alignment of beautiful white teeth but without gums around and between them, demolishes the smile. The image appears like out of a horror movie!

This explains why dentists are always more concerned about your gums than your teeth. Gums are "Impossible to Fix".

6. Overcrowding

Crowding causes many teeth to overlap each other, this creates an oral environment where:
1. It encourages bacteria and food to become trapped between teeth.
2. It is difficult to keep the teeth clean.
3. It encourages tooth decay and gum disease.
4. It is corrected by Orthodontic Treatment.
5. Orthodontic treatment contributes to a lifetime of good oral health and beauty.

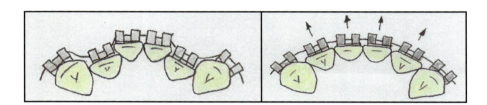

THE WIRE STRAIGHTENS THE TEETH.

Wearing Braces.

Few people grow-up to have straight teeth, and even fewer have spare spaces between them; teeth are commonly crowded.

Straightening teeth is by far the most important step towards having the perfect teeth. Straight teeth generally collect less food, bacteria and stains between them and are easier to be kept clean. This advantage reduces the chances of having decay and gum disease. The smile looks better, the teeth and gums are healthier, the biting is far more comfortable, and with less food trapped between them after each meal, one wouldn't always need to scramble for a toothpick. There is generally less trouble with teeth after orthodontic treatment and wearing braces is an important part of growing up.

Evolution.

Teeth overcrowding is a result of human evolution. As modern diets had become softer less chewing is needed, so humans now have smaller jaws. As a result, without enough space in the mouth for the 32 human adult teeth we had acquired, it often becomes necessary that some of the teeth are extracted in order for the rest to become straight. Few people do have naturally straight teeth, in which case they won't need this treatment. This depends on the size of their teeth in proportion to the size of their jaws, as they had been acquired from their parents. Therefore, a person with large jaws and small teeth could just balance it.

Canines Often Get Left Out.

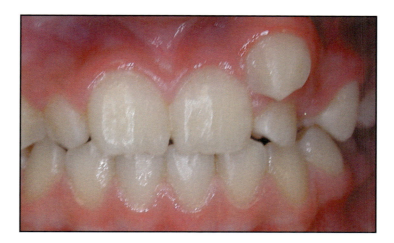

A canine grows high up in the gums.

The canines erupt into the mouth later than most of the teeth around them. As a result they have no space to grow into and so they often grow outside, high up in the gums, or get stuck inside. As canines are very important teeth, and we all have only 4 of them, they should best be retained. They form the four corners of the smile and their tips serve to guide the jaws as you chew side to side. In the past, the oddly growing canine was removed because of this but it's singular removal caused a midline shift at the front teeth. The smile had lost symmetry, and the teeth still remained crooked. If one canine is removed, the corresponding canine on the other side should also be removed, to maintain good balance.

Creating Extra Space.

As we have a total of 8 premolar teeth, and they exist behind the canines, 4 of them are now commonly chosen for extraction to relieve the crowding. The canines are next skillfully dragged into their correct places, to the corners of the mouth. Typically 4 premolar teeth extracted are chosen one from each side of the mouth, left and right, upper and lower, in order to maintain the overall balance and symmetry of the smile. As a result of 4 premolars extracted, enough space is created for straightening the rest of the teeth, and 4 premolars yet remain. Once the teeth are straightened, there are no spaces remaining. If all the teeth are purely straightened without tooth extractions, it is technically possible but it would depend upon the size of the teeth and the jaws. If the teeth are very large and the jaws are moderate or too small, one could end up with a really huge smile ! The teeth could all literally bulge out of the lips right in front of the face, and the smile is too wide. Typically after this treatment, the teeth would tend to collapse back into their crowded positions over time. This is known as a relapse. A good smile is not just about the teeth being straight, but it has to also appear in proportion with the rest of the face. Symmetry and proportionality is indeed the basis for beauty; however beauty is subjective and sometimes what is technically incorrect could turn out to be attractive.

Best Timing-11-13 yrs. Old

Although some corrections may be needed at younger ages for specific minor problems, using removable braces, in general the best time to start orthodontics is when all of the baby teeth have shed, at about the age of 11-13. At this young age all teeth can be moved quickly and easily into their ideal positions. Individual brackets are fixed onto the fronts of teeth to act as handles and a wire passes through them all. These are known as fixed braces. As teeth are safely moved at no more than 1mm per month, the whole process may take 18 months or longer. It is always an advantage to have this treatment done at this age because the results are often better. Braces are also most socially acceptable during childhood.

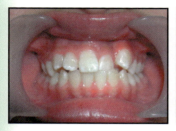
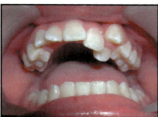
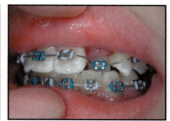
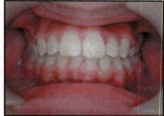

The Shape Of Your Jaws Determines The Shape Of Your Face.

Orthodontic treatment concerns not only with tooth displacement problems but has rather alot to do with dentofacial orthopaedics as it is also involved with controlling the growth of the jaws for obtaining the best bite and aesthetic face profile.

The jaws and teeth are measured and treatments are devised to result in you having them in the best possible positions in your head. This includes a facial symmetry, a straight smile, and the most perfect bite. Results are often dramatic and very pleasing.

Jaw growth control is only possible during childhood. Additional appliances are worn to influence the growth of the jaws in conjunction with the straightening of the teeth. This can result in balanced jaw sizes positioned for an ideal bite, a good smile and also good face and lip profiles. Good biting creates comfort for the jawjoints, and the chewing is efficient and balanced.

Incorrect biting can lead to jawjoint pains and discomforts. The jaws can even click at every time the mouth opens or closes.

Appearances of the smile is always that much better when the jaws and teeth are all correctly positioned. After the jaws had fully grown at the end of adolescence, any correction of their unfavourable shapes and sizes can still be achieved by methods of complex surgery (orthognathic surgery) performed by specialist oral surgeons. The correction of jaws and teeth remains a most influential factor for dramatically improving one's facial appearance.

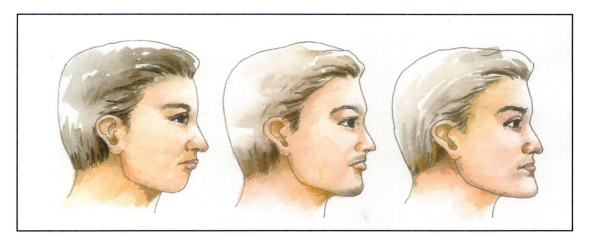

FACIAL PROFILES

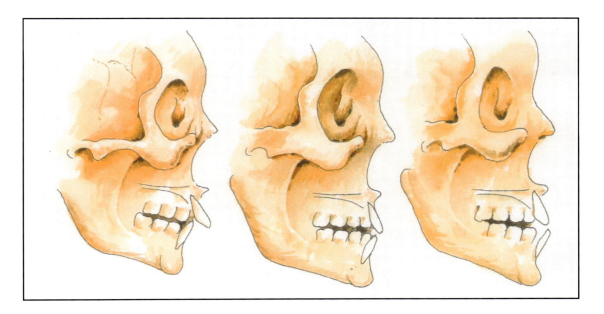

JAW PATTERNS

RETRUDED NORMAL PROTRUDED

PROCEDURE
1. The teeth are generally checked for Orthodontic assesment, then study models and x-rays are taken for treatment planning.
2. Photographs are also usually taken.
3. If teeth need to be extracted, they are planned for extraction in 2 separate visits. (2 premolar teeth removed at each visit).
4. The braces are then fitted onto the teeth at a next visit.
5. Regular monthly or bi-monthly visits to change wires and elastics for the next 18 months/up.
6. At the end of treatment when the teeth are completely straight, the braces are removed. However as the teeth are in their new positions, they are not stable and tend to move back into their wrong positions. This is prevented by wearing retainers.

Things You Should Know About Teeth

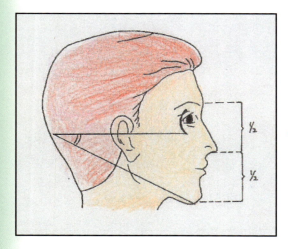

FACIAL PROPORTIONS (THE MOUTH FORMS ONE THIRD OF THE FACE).

What is a headgear?

Sometimes the upper front teeth are sticking out too far forwards and they need to be moved back. Now to connect the elastics to the back teeth, used as anchorage, to pull them back may risk pulling the back teeth forwards, as like a "tug-of-war".

In such instances, it is not a bad idea to use the "back of the head" to provide extra anchorage and hence a headgear is worn.

"In other words, headgear holds back the upper back teeth which in turn pull back the front ones".

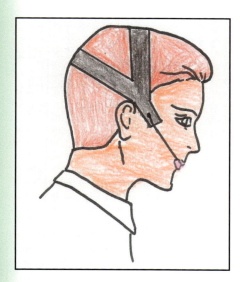   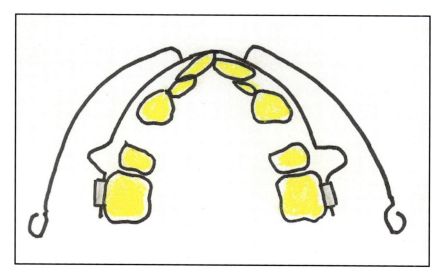

A HEADGEAR   A FACEBOW

The elastic strap of the headgear is connected to the ends of the facebow which slots into the upper brace and reinforces the anchorage for the back teeth. This prevents them from moving forwards as they in turn connect elastics to the front teeth to pull them back. This is known as Extra-oral traction. Without the headgear, as the back teeth pull the front teeth backwards, the back teeth are simultaneously pulled forwards, as like a tug-of-war. Headgear is worn at least for 8 hours everyday, but mostly during sleeping.

Retainers.

When all the teeth are straight and beautiful, the brackets and wires are completely removed. Now the teeth are in their new positions and are likely to be looser and unstable. They all have a tendency to shift back into their original positions, known as a relapse, and it takes a long time for the bone around them to grow strong enough to keep them there. Retainers are provided and they serve to "hold the teeth steady" in their new and perfect positions and these must be worn full-time for the next 2 years for at least 8 hours a day, (during sleep) everyday. There are various types of retainers, some are fixed and some are removable.

All for a good cause.

The straightening of teeth is done once for life and can have by far the most dramatic improvement for one's appearance, forming the most important foundation for a beautiful smile. The health of the teeth and gums always benefit from this treatment. Orthodontic treatment is the one most important procedure offering lifetime benefits which is always worth the time and efforts, but it is unfortunately commonly the one treatment which is often missed with lifelong regrets. It is important to note that during the many months of wearing brackets, brushing is more demanding with the increased accumulation of dental plaque around so many brackets and wires in the mouth, and flossing is not possible. Adults who wish to have their teeth straightened must have any gum diseases completely corrected beforehand because wearing braces can make matters worse in this respect. Children must be very cooperative during the many months of treatment, or else their failure to turn up to their scheduled appointments, failure to perform their daily duties like changing elastics, wearing their headgear, or wearing other accessory gadgets, could seriously delay, or jeopardize the whole exercise.

7. Dental Cavities

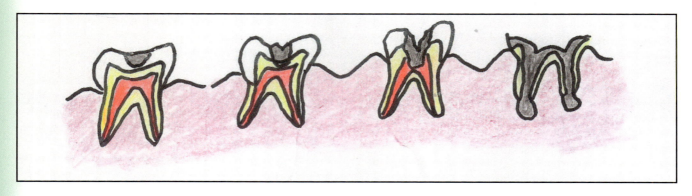

What Is It ?

Also known as dental caries, tooth decay or just cavities, is a most common disease caused by bacteria which damages the structure of teeth causing toothache and infection. This is what causes us to have all our fillings! It affects approximately 90% of schoolchildren worldwide and also most adults, and it causes the most tooth losses in both children and adults. It causes permanent damages to teeth, and always begins as a small hole. If left untreated, the decay penetrates through the entire thickness of enamel, dissolve through dentine, and opens the way for bacteria to infect the nerves within the tooth (dental pulp). This is the common trigger for a major toothache, and when the infection emerges out of the tips of the roots and into the jawbone, it can form a painful abscess. From there the bacteria can spill into the bloodstream to accumulate in other body organs, for example the heart. Although it is very rare, in certain countries some people do die as a result of cavities, even today.

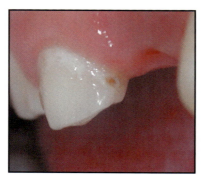 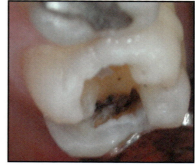

       A Small Hole   A Cavity.

First Signs.

1. The tooth is sensitive to hot, cold and sweet foods.
2. The tooth appears chalky or even grey.
3. Later, the tooth feels slightly throbbing.
4. The tooth throbs a lot with pain, and even wakes you up at night.

Whilst you are unable to see your dentist, try to keep the tooth as clean as possible with your toothbrush. It is sometimes useful to use a mouthwash with fluoride for the time being, but make an appointment as soon as possible. Avoid sweets completely.

Never place a painkiller, especially aspirin, on the gum right next to the painful tooth. It will burn your gums to form a huge, painful ulcer!! This is a very common mistake and placing an aspirin on the side of the tooth doesn't relieve the toothache.

How Does It Work ?

Tooth decay is caused by the organic acids (lactic acid) formed by bacteria in plaque (Streptococcus Mutans) as they ferment the common sugar and refined carbohydrates from our diets, and these acids dissolve the structures of our teeth, initially forming tiny holes for bacteria to enter and rot our teeth. Plaque on the teeth factory the acids, and is fueled by the sugar. (Without the factory, the fuel is harmless on its own).

Brushing all the plaque off the teeth is the ideal way to eliminate tooth decay, but it is easier said than done, especially with young children. The next method is to eliminate all sugar from our diets, in essence to starve the bacteria, but this is even more impossible today. Another way is to substitute the common sugar such as sucrose, with xylitol. In some countries this was successfully done and eating foods with xylitol eliminated sucrose from the equation and reduced tooth decay by up to 90%.

Xylitol

Xylitol, is a natural five-carbon sugar obtained from birch trees and cannot be fermented by plaque to produce acids. Foods which had been made with xylitol, instead of the usual sucrose, glucose, fructose, lactose, galactose, do not cause tooth decay. Chewing xylitol gum 5-30 minutes after a sweet meal serves to prevent tooth decay mostly because its sweetness is harmless, and the action of chewing itself stimulates the increase in salivary flow which washes away your dessert. Saliva is protective, it contains antibodies and also buffers the organic acids. The same increase of salivary flow also occurs with chewing paper, or anything, but xylitol gum is "harmlessly sweet" and tastes better.

Prevention Measures.

1. Fluoride

"Teeth exposed to fluoride in the first 18 years of life reduced cavities by up to 50% and it maintains their increased resistance to decay throughout life."

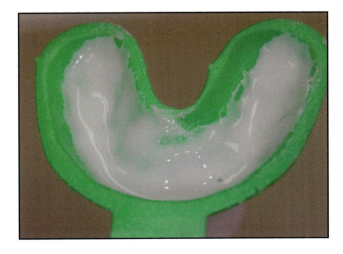

Fluoride gel is delivered in a disposable mouth-tray.

Tooth decay causes unnecessary pain and suffering and is nowadays considered a very preventable disease with thanks to the discovery of fluoride. The protection for teeth offered by this mineral had made a major impact on the reduction of tooth decay worldwide. Fluoride combines with the tooth structure to form a much harder structure which resists dissolution by acid attacks. New teeth in the mouth are weaker with lower mineral contents and are easily dissolved by organic acids. Teeth were never meant to face the excess amounts of sugar nowadays in our modern diets but before they have time to take up more calcium from the saliva to get strong, they are already bathed in plaque and sweets .

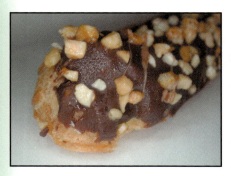 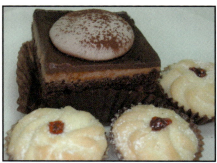 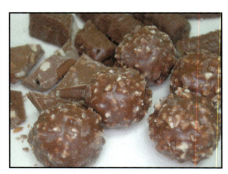

Fluoride has become a major discovery in the history of dentistry. Topical fluoride treatment for teeth done at the dental clinic once or twice a year benefits young children particularly, and the most practical time to begin it is around the age of 3.

More About Fluoride.

Fluoride is effective because it discourages plaque accumulation on tooth surfaces, it is antibacterial and discourages the bacteria to ferment organic acids. It encourages calcium from the saliva to deposit back into the decayed tooth surfaces and it discourages the calcium to be dissolved from the teeth by the acids. Fluoride incorporated into the calcium structure of teeth is rendered more resistant to dissolution by acid attacks. Excess intake of fluoride is perhaps toxic, but rare, and it could only be achieved by actually swallowing large amounts of it. This could happen if fluoride tablets were over-prescribed and swallowed at a young age, or swallowed by mothers during pregnancy. So long as the dosages are carefully prescribed, there are advantages of ingesting fluoride in an attempt to strengthen the teeth before they erupt. Children under the age of 6 who inadvertently swallow tubes of fluoridated toothpastes or gallons of highly fluoridated drinking water could perhaps develop vomiting, diarrhea and get fluorosis of the teeth, a condition when teeth become permanently darkly stained and speckled, but this event is highly unlikely. Fluoride tablets and drops are perhaps advantageous but the dosages must be monitored very professionally. The most effective time for swallowing prescribed fluoride tablets or drops is below the age of 6. However it is less popular nowadays and the topical application of fluoride is considered safer and is widely preferred.

2. Fissure Sealants For Molars

"A single application of fissure sealants on molar teeth can provide remarkable protection for the fissures of back teeth."

Adult molar teeth are at great risks for tooth decay mainly because they have naturally deep fissures within their chewing surfaces which collect and stagnate bacteria and sugary foods. Biscuits, chocolate, cakes and such snacks are plunged inside and are never well washed out by the tongue afterwards. The fissure sealant, is a plastic resin which flows and fills into all the fissures and harden inside, sealing these crevices for good. No drilling is necessary for this procedure. As soon as the "1st adult molar tooth" erupts into the mouth at about the age of 6, they are best fissure-sealed immediately.

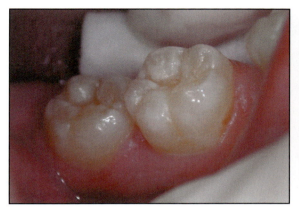 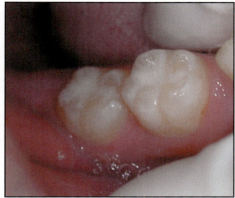

DEEP PITS AND FISSURES   FISSURE SEALANTS

FISSURE SEALANTS ARE BEST APPLIED ON THESE FIRST MOLAR ADULT TEETH JUST AFTER THEY APPEAR IN THE MOUTH ABOUT THE AGE OF 6.

Words Of Advice.

We know that refined carbohydrates and the common sugar causes tooth decay, but it is not so much the quantity of these consumed at each meal that damages teeth, rather it has more to do with the frequency of sugary snacks during each day that determines the multiple damage attack episodes. Sticky sweets are especially bad because they stick around for too long, and the prolonged bottle-feeding to a child is disastrous because the constant bathing for hours would cause damage to every tooth. The worst thing to do for children is to allow them to suck on a bottle during their sleep. This will result in rampant and indiscriminant tooth decay to occur on every tooth and at their every surfaces and it is a condition also known as bottle-caries. It is worth remembering that even milk contains hidden sugars, amongst others. Saliva must be given time between each meal to wash and neutralize any acids on the teeth. Never have any snacks just before bedtime because salivary flow is reduced during sleep. Brushing teeth just before sleeping is an ideal habit. It is always a good idea to rinse the mouth with water after every meal. Whenever you eat out, there is always a glass of water provided. Make it a habit to take a last sip of it just before you leave.

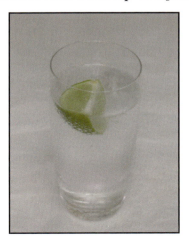

Treatment
Facing The Drill !

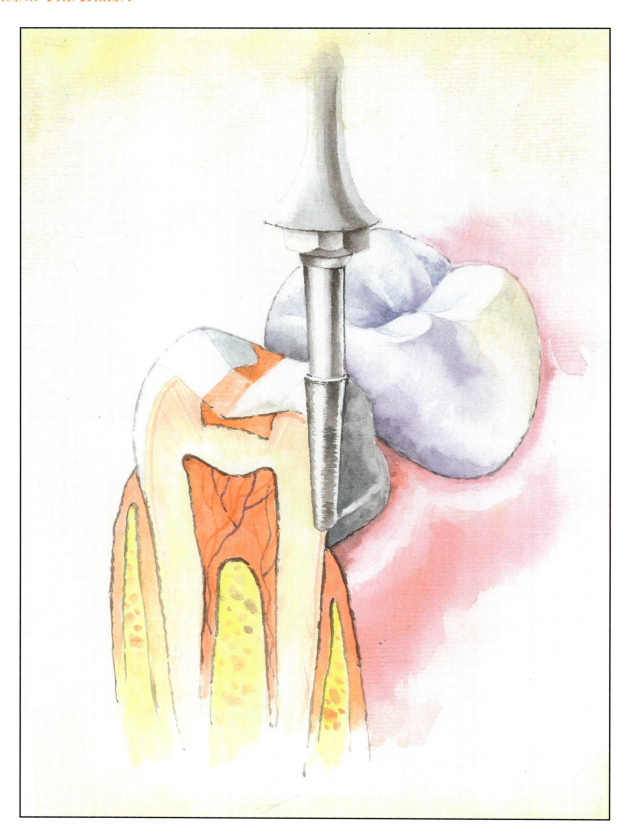

Once you have a cavity, you would need a filling. If you are terrified of water splashing into your mouth during the procedure, you may request your dentist to put on a rubber-dam on the tooth before he starts. The rubber-dam will isolate your tooth and it prevents water from entering your throat.

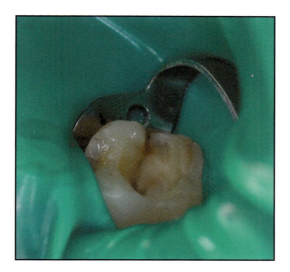

You may also request to have an anaesthetic gel to be applied to the gums which numbs up the gum surface in 3 minutes before you have the injection. This way you won't quite feel "the jab".

SMALL FILLINGS

Composite resins, also known as white fillings, are commonly used to restore the small cavities in the front teeth. They have a good range of colours, and blend well with the tooth. It is a kind of hard plastic filling. The dentist will first drill away all the decay in your cavity. The cavity is then acid treated for a few seconds, washed and dried, and the composite resin is flowed in.

Acid treatment allows the resin to superglue with the tooth. A light then shines on the white filling for about 40 seconds and hardens it. It is then polished.

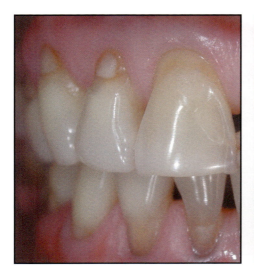 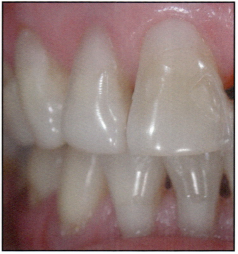

Amalgams, are the commonly used silver-black coloured metal fillings for restoring the holes in the back teeth. It contains approximately 50% of mercury, mixed with copper, silver, tin and zinc. Mercury amalgam had existed for centuries and used in dentistry because it is cheap, durable and considered safe despite its high mercury content. Mercury is of course a very potent neurotoxin and there is still an on-going debate regarding the absolute certainty of its safety since amalgam fillings have been shown to increase mercury blood levels. For it to be harmless to the human body during its decades of existence in the mouth is not guaranteed. It is currently considered safe until proven otherwise because it had already been in use for decades.

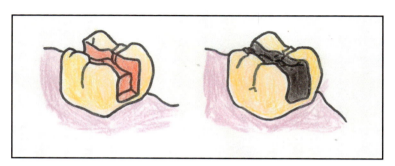
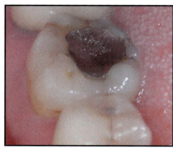

Amalgam Filling
Fillings Should Be Polished.

Whereas composite resin fillings harden enough to be polished in the same visit, amalgam fillings are soft to begin with and require up to 24 hours to attain its full strength, and so it cannot be polished until the day after when it has fully hardened. It is very good practice to return to your dentist to have amalgam fillings polished. This takes only 2 minutes without need for injections, making the amalgam smooth and shiny like your precious silverware. They are more hygienic and can be kept cleaner. Unpolished fillings are often rough and pitted collecting a lot of dental plaque and black stains. Polishing amalgam fillings can help to prolong their longevity and improves the overall oral hygiene. A good amalgam filling can last for 10 years or more if it is fairly small. They are expected to require replacement once they have deteriorated.

Composites resins and amalgams are soft when placed into the cavities, but harden later. They are quick to do, and also cheaper because they do not require to be made at the dental laboratory. However they can also distort in shape after years in the mouth, staining and deteriorating at their edges. Sometimes amalgams can break up into many pieces after years of chewing on them.

Larger Fillings
Cast Fillings-inlays.

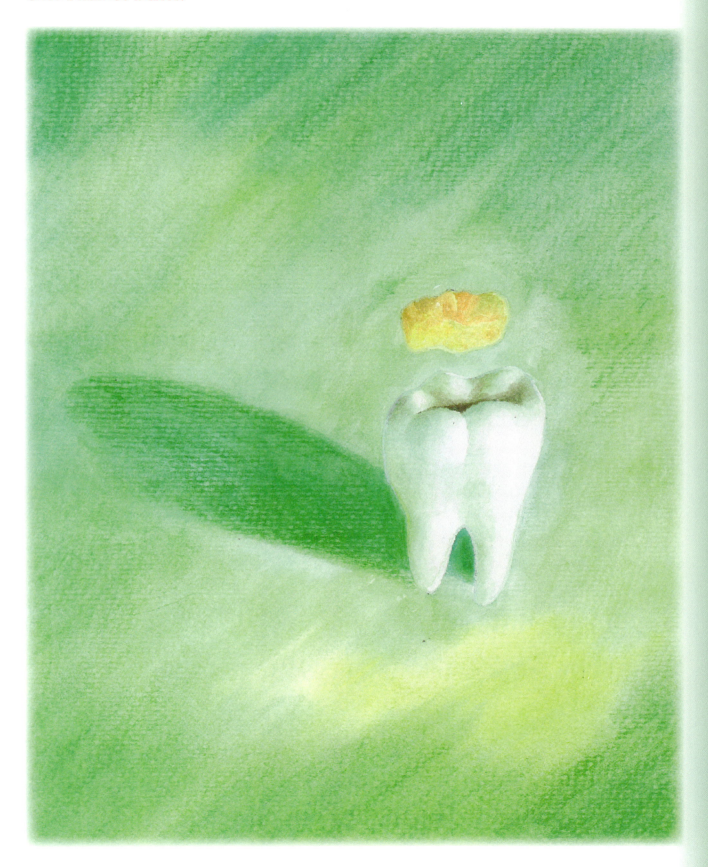

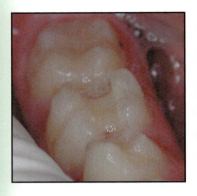
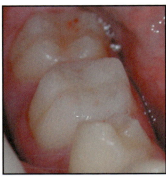

Porcelain Filling (Inlay)

Inlays are custom made cast fillings, hardened and ready to fit into your larger cavities. In general they last longer but are more expensive to make. They are typically of gold, non-precious metals or porcelain, and each individual inlay is to be constructed at the dental laboratory from a model of your cavity. Apart from filling your hole, inlays have better anatomical shapes to mimic your lost tooth cusps for better biting and chewing. This treatment thus requires two separate visits.

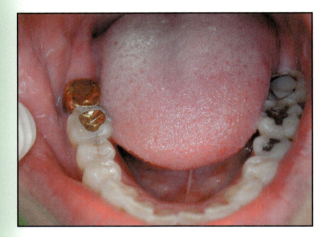
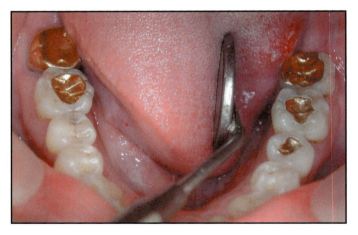

Gold fillings (inlays) always tend to last better than amalgams. It is a good idea to replace old amalgams with gold inlays.

Dental Cavities

Material Choices.

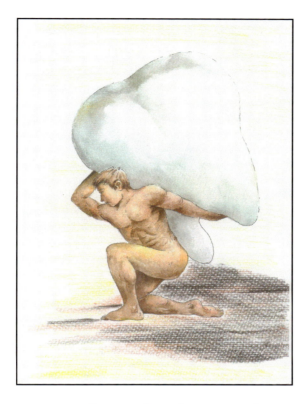

Materials used to restore your damaged teeth are very important and can determine the length of time it can protect your tooth. If the filling material itself crumbles in time after years of chewing, there will be leakages for decay to recur inside. Generally speaking the smaller the filling, the longer they last, for any given material. However, it becomes more critical when the cavity is very large. An amalgam will not remain unaltered after years of chewing. It can deform or fracture after several years to create leakages. Gold on the other hand, can remain mostly unaltered for decades, and can provide a better service than amalgam.

1. Pure gold or 24K, is too soft for chewing and so an alloy of gold with other metals such as platinum, palladium, silver and copper to increase their hardness. Such gold fillings and crowns in 18K or 14K, have excellent durability, wear well, and unlike porcelain, does not excessively wear the opposing teeth. Gold had always been considered the benchmark of all materials because they cast accurately, and are less likely to tarnish and corrode, and as a result it is not uncommon for a gold filling to last well for 30 years in the mouth.
2. Porcelain is beautiful, but can be very abrasive to the natural tooth it bites on. The other concern is that it can fracture.
3. Cheaper metals like silver-palladium alloys (white gold) and nickel-chromium alloys both have problems with shrinkages after casting, and their fitting with the tooth is less accurate. They are more prone to corrosion and tarnishing. These fillings will leak as a result, inviting decay back into the cavity they served to protect.

A Word About Dental Porcelains.

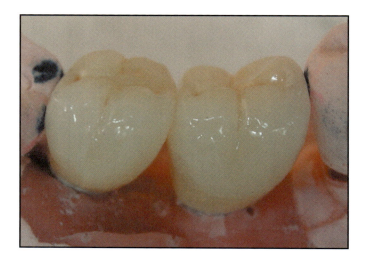

The ceramic material known as "porcelain", holds a special place in dentistry, producing aesthetically pleasing results.

Their colour, translucency and vitality remains unmatched by all other materials in the profession. This material dates back to the 17thCentury from China and it was not until 1838, that Elias Wildman, produced dental porcelain with the translucency and shades that reasonably matched natural teeth. The earliest porcelains were mixtures of Kaolin, Feldspar and Quartz.

Composition Of Modern Dental Porcelains.

Modern dental porcelains today are mainly feldspathic glass with crystalline inclusions of silica-feldspars, and are mixtures of: **POTASSIUM ALUMINIUM SILICATE – $K_2O \cdot Al_2O_3 \cdot 6SiO_2$**
+ **SODIUM ALUMINIUM SILICATE (or, ALBITE)-$Na_2O \cdot Al_2O_3 \cdot 6SiO_2$**
+ **QUARTZ**

Since the discovery, by Buonocore in 1955, that enamel could be modified for the purpose of its bonding, porcelains may now be bonded to enamel and dentine in this way. However the flexural strengths of porcelains remain a concern as they are prone to fracturing under stress. Porcelains are basically rigid and brittle, whose strengths are also reduced by the presence of internal voids and porosities.

There Are 2 Ways To Compensate For This:
1. **Metal Supporting Structures.**

The weaker porcelains are partially compensated by means of metal supporting structures, i. e. metal backings. With this inclusion, the crowns could become bulbous and tremendous skill is involved to keep them slim.

For This Purpose-

- gold alloys, high (75%), medium (50%), low golds (2%) are all suitable.

-silver-palladium alloys (white golds) can tarnish under the porcelain because of the high silver content, and if they blacken, it is rather like wearing a black swimsuit under a white shirt, and the tooth will look overall, grey; in addition, the casting shrinkages, and resulting poor-fittings are

less forgiving leading to eventual failure by leakages which cause recurrent decay.

-nickel-chromium alloys are the cheapest and most popular, but have problems of bonding weakest to the porcelain.

Nickel is not biocompatible, and some people are known to have allergies to this metal.

They also have the highest casting shrinkage for a poorest-fit, inviting leakages for recurrent decay.

2. Inserting Alumina- "Aluminous Porcelains"

Although the full range of dental porcelains today are all aesthetically pleasing, they differ immensely in terms of their flexural strengths, ranging from values of 60 to 120 mpa at one end, and up to 687 mpa (comparable to metals) at the other, the latter being made up of a dense-sintered aluminium oxide. Adding powdered alumina can achieve its significant strengthening, alumina particles act as the "crack-stoppers" preventing the propagation of a crack when the tooth is under stress. However this aluminous structure is rather opaque, it is often used as the core, or inner layer, of the crown, to serve as an underlying backing for the superficial layer of less dense, but far more aesthetic porcelain. Aesthetically, porcelain is an almost perfect material for the replacement of absent tooth substances. It provides a spectrum of shades and translucencies, and can be layered with craftsmanship to achieve an almost life-like appearance. Translucencies may be added for the tips of the teeth for more realism. Unlike metals, which are uncosmetic for the visible areas of the mouth, porcelain is suitable for every tooth restoration in the mouth and is nowadays, a popular favourite. Additionally, porcelain is considered biocompatible.

Crowns

When the cavity in a tooth is too large, the wall of the cavity may become too thin to hold any material inside, and so a crown is needed. Crowns are often made of full gold, full porcelain, or porcelain fused to gold or to metal (for strength), or simply metal. The tooth is filed down circumferentially to allow space for the crown to encase it. A mold is taken and sent to the dental laboratory for fabrication. A temporary crown is normally provided at the end of treatment. The colour shades of your natural teeth are selected if the crown is to be made of porcelain, and a second appointment is scheduled for its cementation after the crown is made.

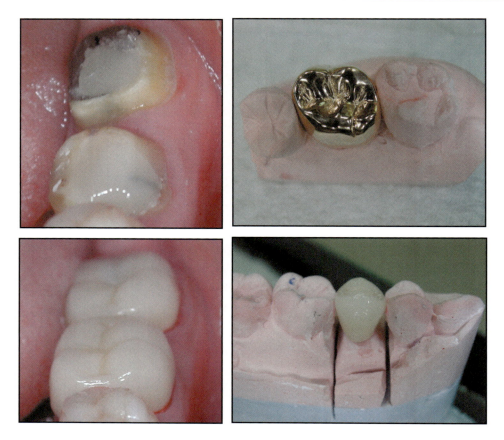

Crowns entirely made of porcelain, or porcelain jacket crowns look more natural and beautiful for the front teeth as they allow natural light to pass straight through them and into dentine. This translucency gives them a more life-like appearance.

The criteria is that the porcelain must be adequately strengthened with densely packed aluminium oxide to resist fracturing.

This is why a good quality porcelain jacket crown is often more expensive.

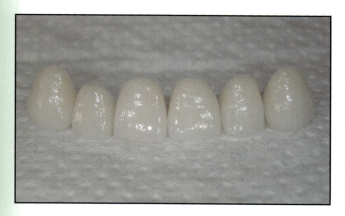   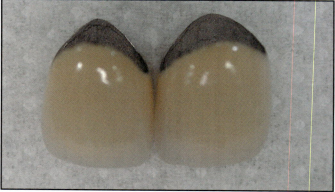

PORCELAIN JACKET CROWNS   **PORCELAIN BONDED TO METAL CROWNS**

PORCELAIN JACKET CROWNS LOOK MORE LIFE-LIKE THAN PORCELAIN BONDED TO METAL CROWNS, WHICH APPEAR DULLER AND MORE LIFELESS.

However they are less suitable for the back teeth because they could fracture with heavy biting. Gold or metal crowns are best for the back teeth if they are not readily visible. Methods to combine gold or metal for strength, with porcelain for whiteness, known as porcelain-bonded crowns have become very successful for back teeth. These are basically gold or metal crowns covered with and outside layer of porcelain and because it gives the best of both worlds, it has become a popular combination. However, people who have a tendency to grind their teeth are best advised to avoid porcelain completely and to have their back teeth restored in gold.

How Long Do They Last?

Everything is determined by the level of your oral hygiene. The most worrying factor is the recurrence of decay around all fillings and crowns. However, if well cared for, good quality crowns are expected to last beyond 15 years and up to 30 years.

Good cast fillings can enjoy the same level of durability. Basic direct fillings such as the amalgams and composite resins do appear to last for 10-12 years, but so long as they are small. These are limited by their inherent material weakness and do tend to deteriorate over time, but they are cheap. If anything, they are good value for the money, but they do have their time limits.

Root Canal Treatment.

If bacteria has infected the nerve, root canal treatment will be necessary to save the tooth and an anaesthetic injection is needed. The bacteria grows and multiplies in the infected nerve and these will eventually emerge from the tooth at the tips of their roots to produce painful abscesses, right underneath. At the same time the whole root structure will rot on the inside without causing any pain. The nerve tissues and blood vessels also become rotten flesh which could smell very nasty. Root canal treatment removes these and also the decay inside, cleaning out everything within the entire lengths of the root canals.

Root canal treatment is needed if the pulp dies from whatever reason, whether it is caused by tooth decay or involved in extensive tooth fractures. The treatment is very tedious and involves removing all the nerve, blood vessels and bacteria inside. The canals are cleaned with special files and as all the nerves are interconnected as one complex, the entire network must be removed. The inside of the tooth is copiously flushed with distilled water and then disinfected with an antiseptic dressing placed inside the tooth at the end of the first treatment and a temporary filling is used to seal the cavity. 2-3 visits are often needed to control the infection. Some discomforts may occur during the initial stages and the tooth may be tender to bite on. This would subside after the infection had cleared. Pain killers and antibiotic medicines are often also prescribed. Subsequent visits are painless and may not require an anaesthetic. The canals are then all finally sealed with a material called gutta percha.

STEP 1. ALL THE DECAY IN THE CAVITY IS REMOVED BY THE DRILL.
STEP 2. A FILE IS USED TO CLEAN OUT EVERYTHING INSIDE, RIGHT DOWN TO THE BOTTOM.
STEP 3. THE TOOTH IS FLUSHED AND DRIED WITH DISPOSABLE ABSORBANT PAPER-POINTS.
STEP 4. AN ANTISEPTIC MEDICINE IS PLACED INSIDE THE TOOTH AND SEALED TEMPORARILY.
STEP 5. FINALLY GUTTA PERCHA IS USED TO PERMANENTLY SEAL THE ENTIRE

INSIDES OF THE ROOT.

It is important that the whole tooth is completely sealed inside from top to bottom or else any voids within the tooth could allow the bacteria inside to grow and cause all the insides to rot. The filling or crown must also provide a water-tight seal.

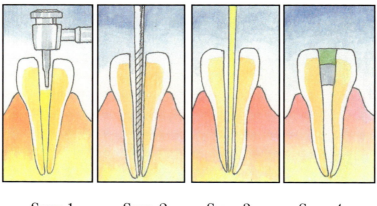

STEP 1.   STEP 2.   STEP 3.   STEP 4.

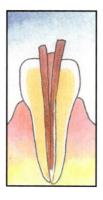

STEP 5.

STEP 6. Teeth which had been extensively damaged by tooth decay and treated by this method are rather weaker. They are brittle and are often ready to crumble with a heavy bite, (especially if it is a back tooth), and a crown is certainly needed.

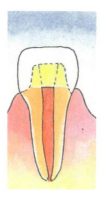

STEP 6.

8. Self-inflicted Wear

1. Attrition, abrasion, erosion
2. Most people are unaware of it.
3. Many teeth are damaged at the same time.
4. Treatment often involves repairing too many teeth

Bad Habits.

Apart from tooth decay and gum disease, we often forget that we might be doing our own damage unknowingly by ourselves.

It might be inevitable that teeth will have wear and tear after decades of service, but some people adopt habits which significantly accelerate their wear. This type of self-damage is very extensive as it involves many teeth simultaneously.

Although enamel is the hardest tooth structure in the body, and feels no pain, one is never aware of it until it is too late.

As enamel is white, but the dentine is yellow, enamel worn thin will allow the yellow dentine to become more apparent, making the tooth looking yellow. This is one reason why teeth appear more yellow as we age.

1. ATTRITION is the wearing of teeth by heavy grinding. "Don't grind your teeth !"

Did you know that a person could exert up to 25kg of force on his teeth, for 2 seconds at a time during each grind?

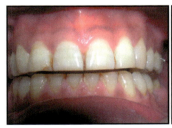
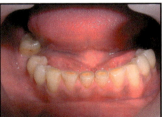
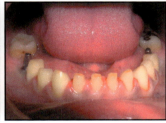
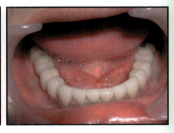

Attrition Wear

BRUXISM: This is an oral para-functional activity and most people do have this behaviour to varying extents unknowingly.

It involves clenching and grinding of the teeth and alot of us do it all the time without thinking. Some people do it during sleep via reflexes controlled by the brain. Even when the brain control is switched off during sleep, this reflex activity continues and this is known as night bruxism. Teeth grinding can be so loud that it can often wake the spouse up during the night, and pain at the jawjoints are also felt the next morning. The jaw muscles also become tender with aches. This condition is often associated with stress. In this way the teeth are eventually all worn down, flat and short. This damage is permanent !

The only best solution is to make crowns for every worn tooth in order to replace the abraded and lost tooth tissues, restoring teeth back to their original forms. Wearing nightguards during sleep will not stop bruxism but it prevents damage to the teeth during, and will also provide some comfort for the jawjoints.

2. **ABRASION** is the wearing of teeth by devices such as a toothbrush. Toothbrush abrasion is a most common damage caused by over-enthusiastic toothbrushing. People who need to smile a lot in their occupation tend to wear their teeth in this way.

Little do they realize afterwards that it does more harm than good. The teeth appears yellow because after the white enamel is worn the dentine underneath shows through. Scrubbing teeth too hard recedes the gums and exposes the necks of the teeth, showing their bare roots! Exposed dentine is very sensitive and respond painfully to hot and cold, so painful it is commonly confused with decay. Composite resin fillings can be used to restore cavities caused by abrasion, but the receded gums will remain permanently. There are also varnishes that the dentist can apply to block the sensitivities. However, once the teeth are abraded no longer, and the habit ceases, the sensitivities usually subside naturally. Toothpastes for sensitivities are also useful.

Toothbrushing is good, but it does cause some tooth wear in the long term. It is important to strike a balance and be able to remove the soft dental plaque lightly whilst at the same time it does not cause too much tooth wear.

Plaque is fairly soft and is readily removed without heavy scrubbings. Composite resin fillings can be used to restore cavities caused by abrasion, but the receded gums will remain with you permanently. There is no effective method to grow the gums back down again. Using a soft toothbrush is more gentle on the teeth and a light but thorough brushing technique in circular or up and down movements is always preferable. Electric toothbrushes are nowadays popular, and best for people who are just heavy-handed with their manual toothbrushes. Their light movements reduces your tendencies to wear your teeth quickly. Some people can spend a full 15 minutes each time they brush their teeth, and over time, this is the result. It becomes a kind of obsession, or paranoia!

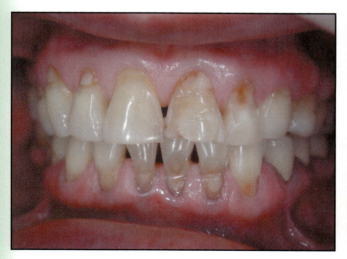 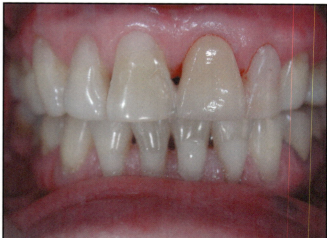

Abrasion Wear

3. **EROSION** is the slow dissolving of teeth by acidic foods and drinks. Some people adopt the habit of sucking on citrus fruits like grapefruits and lemons, and this can eventually dissolve

away the enamel and dentine in the long term. Repeated exposure to stomach acids over time can also cause serious erosion of teeth. People with stomach problems frequently regurgitate acids into their mouths would never realize the erosion caused to their teeth, over time. Stomach problems must be treated properly.

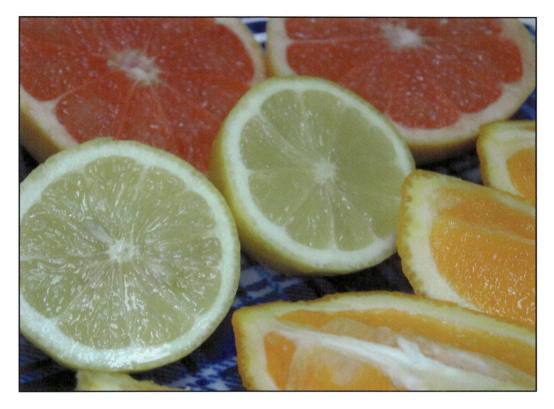

Sucking On Citrus Fruits

4. HABIT CHEWING ON HARD OBJECTS.
Some people enjoy chewing on their pencils, nibble at their fingernails, and they bite on all sorts of hard objects.
Chewing animal bones and the shells of crabs and lobsters cause teeth to chip and break. This is very common.

9. Wisdom Teeth

1. Causes irreparable damages to the tooth in front of it.
2. Causes serious infections in the mouth and face.
3. Commonly impacted.
4. Prone to tooth decay.
5. Best extracted early if advised.

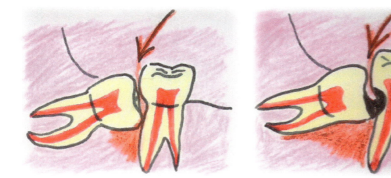

Wisdom teeth are the last teeth to erupt in the mouth, usually between the ages of 17 to 25, which is why they are commonly stuck! They are the 3rd molar teeth at the back of the mouth and are difficult to be cleaned. Most people have four wisdom teeth but some people have less, and the very lucky few have none. If the mouth is small, they may fail to appear at all and can remain deep but dormant inside the jawbones. X-rays taken by the dentist can confirm their forms, positions and existence . If deeply embedded in the jaws without the contamination of saliva and food, they usually never cause any problems. However, they must be checked regularly with x-rays because on very rare occasions, cysts could develop around them. If wisdom teeth had erupted into good and upright positions, are functioning normally, and are able to be kept clean there is no reason to extract them. However, they are prone to decay if the brushing slips, and so if you have decided to keep your wisdom teeth, make brushing at them your first priority before you brush the rest of the mouth. It may be helpful for you to use a baby toothbrush for this sole purpose.

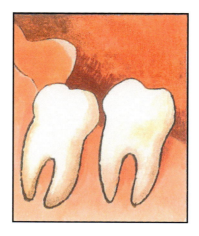

Most commonly there is only a partial space in the mouth for it and gets trapped under a gum-flap to impact against the molar tooth in front. Food and bacteria wedges between both teeth. This gum-flap tends to swell up with infection, a condition known as pericoronitis and is very painful. The upper wisdom tooth also bites on it readily and this excruciation is by far the commonest reason for prompting an emergency extraction. When it erupts half-way and gets stuck in this manner, it can cause painful infections and become grossly decayed, affecting itself and the molar tooth in front, simultaneously.

About 60% of people had experienced one or more impacted wisdom teeth in their lives, and it was the repeat of infections which commonly prompted their extractions. Infections from wisdom teeth can be very painful and serious. The infection spreads uncontrollably to the face and the swelling can be huge and alarming. Swallowing is difficult, and trismus can develop, (a condition when the mouth cannot open). When this happens, the volume of pus must firstly be drained and the infection controlled before the wisdom tooth could be extracted. Painkillers could never be effective until the infection is successfully controlled, so don't take the risk of delaying the problem with your home tablets! Infections must always be dealt with promptly and professionally. Wisdom teeth infections are like potential time-bombs.

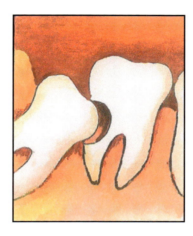

Tooth decay typically also involves the tooth in front as food traps between them. The damage done to both teeth after serious pain is felt is often so late and bad that both are extracted simultaneously.

Home Management Of A Wisdom Tooth Infection.

Analgesics.
Take some pain-killers if necessary, but never place an aspirin tablet over the tooth as it may burn a hole in the gums.
All pain-killers are effective, aspirin, paracetamol, mefenamic acid, ibuprofen, codeine, tylenol(acetaminophen), amongst others.

Hot Salt Mouth Wash (Hsmw).
The frequent use of hot salt mouthwashes, or any antibacterial mouthwashes will help to relieve the discomfort.

Use A Soft Brush To Clean Area.
Keep the area as clean as possible using a soft toothbrush.

Refrain From Smoking Completely As Tobacco Will Worsen The Situation.
See Your Dentist As Soon As Possible.

1.   The choice of tooth extractions under Local or General Anaesthesia.
    In general terms, local anaesthesia by injections at the dental office is by far simpler and safer than "going under" as in general anaesthesia, the latter being more costly, and more risky. If a general anaesthesia is to be given, all the wisdom teeth in the mouth should be removed together during the single session in a private hospital.

2.   Is the tooth to be extracted with forceps, or is a surgery required?
    This depends on the position of the tooth, whether it is upright enough to be grasped readily by the forceps.
    Usually the upper wisdom teeth are uprighted and are removed easily, but not the lower as they are often impacted and grown sideways. Under a local anaesthetic, the gum is lifted and the tooth is separated into fragments, and these are dissected out of the socket. The gum is stitched back into place to cover the wound.

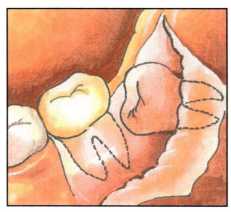 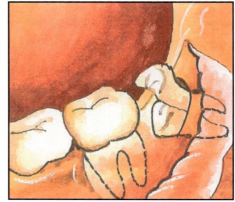

INSTRUCTIONS AFTER WISDOM TEETH EXTRACTIONS.
If you have just had your wisdom teeth removed, please take note of these instructions:

1.   Do not to consume food for at least 30 minutes or so after until the numbness has gone. Be careful not to chew your lip, or take any hot drinks, as you may burn yourself during the lips are still numb. A soft diet to start with is advisable for the first 2 days, but remember to avoid smoking completely.

2. Avoid excessive exercise and alcohol for the remainder of the day as it may initiate bleeding. Do not rinse or cause disturbances to the socket as the clot may become dislodged. The clot acts as a plug in the socket and is important for the healing process. Eat and drink normally, but do not allow food to fall into the socket, but if so, do not attempt to "pick them out" with a toothpick, or bleeding will resume. Some slight traces of blood is expected to trickle initially, but large quantities of bleeding will require professional attention.

Roll up a moistened piece of cotton gauze or hankerchief and bite at it on the bleeding site, or alternatively, moisten and bite onto a used teabag for about 30 minutes or more. If the bleeding persists, call your dentist immediately.

3. Keep the rest of the mouth as clean as possible by routine brushing.

Take the medicines provided as according to their prescription. Painkillers can be ommited if the pain had subsided but the full course of antibiotics prescribed must be taken. Swelling is inevitable the day after surgery but you can place an ice-pack onto the swelling on the face for 15 minutes on and 15 minutes off alternately during the first two days in order to limit the swelling. Once the swelling had maximized by the third day, use a hot towel in the same manner applying it to the face to bring the swelling down.

10. Infections

Infections in the mouth is common as the mouth is full of bacteria. The usual causes for mouth infections are tooth decay, gum disease, and impacted wisdom teeth. Some people are more prone to infections if they have poor oral hygiene, or have less saliva in the mouth because of taking too many medicines. Good health and nutrition also plays a important role for our defense ability against infections. However heavy smokers are also at greater risk of developing oral infections.

Abscess.

Pus discharging from the gums may not be painful when there is no pressure build-up. However when the pus is trapped it forms a "balloon", called an abscess, and it can be painful. If you should realize that you have an abscess, or begin to feel a slight swelling, you must have it checked by your dentist as soon as possible and have it managed early. Hot salt mouth washes are particularly useful in the meantime, but smoking will make things worse. If an abscess exists, the pus could spread further and make things worse. Medicines alone will not work and the pus must be drained at the clinic as soon as possible. This drainage will give you relief immediately. It is absolutely essential to identify the tooth which is causing your infection and you must have it either treated or extracted. Even if an abscess is painless but you do know it is there, you must never hesitate to seek treatment as early as possible. Keeping abscesses in the mouth is not healthy for you and the bacteria can leak into your bloodstream and be carried to other body organs.

Bacteria In The Blood.

The gum line is in fact an open gateway for bacteria to enter into your bloodstream, known as bacteraemia. This is why it is so important to keep your teeth as clean as possible, particularly at the gum line. Unknowingly minute traces of bacteria do enter our bloodstream everyday from our gums at the gum lines. Under normal circumstances, as these traces are indeed minute, our body defenses protect us enough from their harm and we would never fall ill because of it.

Coronary Heart Disease.

There is a direct correlation between gum disease and heart disease and researchers have found that people who have gum disease are twice as likely to develop coronary heart disease. One theory for this is that the bacteria which enters the bloodstream via the gums can travel and infect the already accumulated fat within the coronary artery to damage it further.

Heart Valve Infections.

The heart, and in particular the heart valves are at risk of infection. Those who have already had their heart valves damaged by Rheumatic Fever at childhood are at great risk of becoming infected again during life by the oral bacteria (S. Viridans) and a next attack can cause the fatal condition known as Infective Endocarditis (I. E.). This re-infection is most unaffordable.

It is now thought that their maintaining the highest standard of daily oral hygiene all-year-round is a real life-saver.

People who have had their heart valves damaged before and visit their dentists for a scale and polish or tooth extractions, should have an antibiotic medicine taken orally 1 hour beforehand. Gum disease and abscesses in the mouth should never be tolerated as they can be a good source of bacteria for infecting the heart.

Sinus infections and your upper back teeth

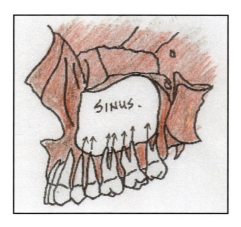

Side View Of The Upper Back Teeth

Did you know that your maxillary sinuses exist just above your upper back teeth. The roots of these teeth are pointing upwards towards these sinuses and sometimes their tips even penetrate right into them. If any upper back teeth should develop an infection, the bacteria and pus can spread from its roots to enter into the sinus directly. This can cause a bacterial sinusitis.

11. Smoking

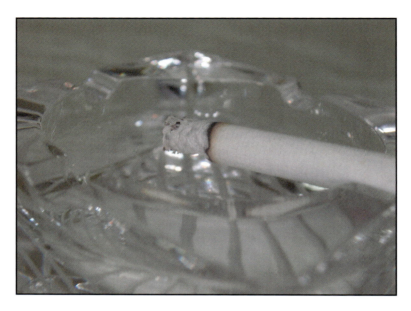

"Worldwide, 47% of men and 12% of women smoke a total of 6 trillion cigarettes a year, and 4 million people die worldwide each year as a result of smoking, as according to a 1999 survey by the World Health Organisation".

Oral Cancer.

Studies have already indicated that there is a definite link between smoking and the development of oral cancer as over 75% of the cases are smokers. Generally in the western world, oral cancer can account for up to 6% of all cancers but it is very dominant in Asia. When smoking is combined with heavy drinking, the risk of oral cancer increases 15 times more than non-smokers. The average 5-year survival rate of patients with oral cancer is about 50%, and this is because they are often discovered very late. The average age for the diagnosis is about 60. Heavy smoking and heavy drinking are lifestyle habits, but when the two combine, they act together synergistically to seriously harm the body.

Signs of oral cancer include white or red patches in the mouth, swellings in the neck, a mouth ulcer under the tongue which never heals. In general, if you have any problems in the mouth which is uncomfortable and does not heal in 2 weeks, they should be checked by your dentist, who may refer you to a specialist for all further investigations. Routine dental check-ups are also important because the dentist could discover and bring these to your attention before it becomes late.

The Mouth.

Smoking also accelerates gum disease, causes more bad breath, and more tartar and stains on your teeth. Smoking in general deteriorates the oral tissues.

12. Dental Trauma

"A Blow To The Face !"
1. Upper front teeth are commonly lost as a result of a childhood accident.
2. Children are particularly vulnerable.
3. Front teeth which stick-out must be corrected early before they get smashed.
4. Mouth guards should always be worn during contact sports.

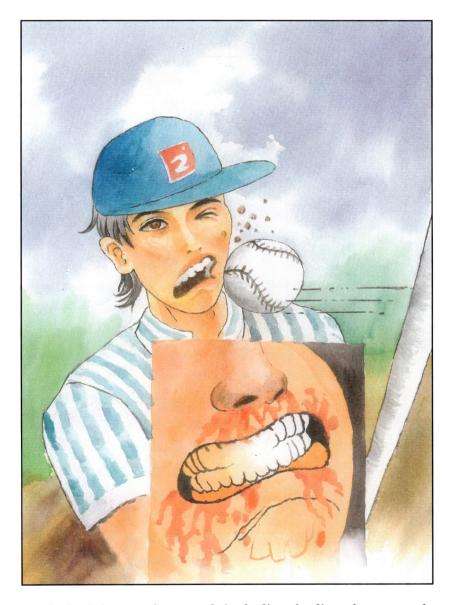

Dental trauma is the injury to the mouth including the lips, the gums, the tongue, the teeth and the jawbones. Quite often the upper two front teeth are either seriously injured or are totally knocked-out! They could be hit either directly by a front blow, or indirectly by the blow to the chin, and are smashed by the lower teeth. The lip or tongue are often bitten in the process. If the teeth were already biting on a mouth guard during the accident the teeth would be protected from each other, and the lips and tongue would be less likely bitten.

THINGS YOU SHOULD KNOW ABOUT TEETH

PROTECTION PROVIDED BY A MOUTHGUARD

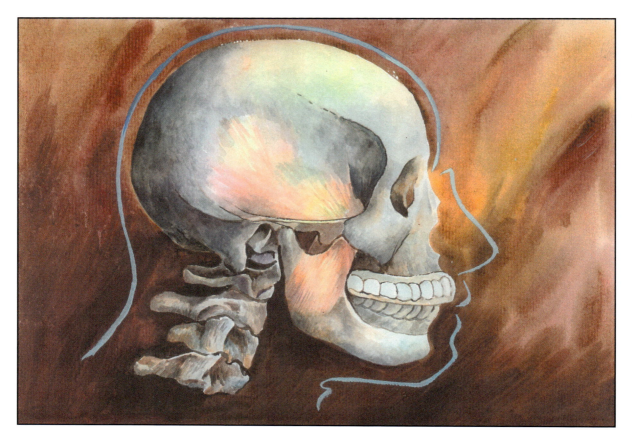

In all contact sports like boxing, ice-hockey, football, and basketball, face-accidents can cause serious damage to the teeth and jaws and the wearing of mouthguards can help to limit the extent of the damage by distributing the impact energy. If the impact hits the chin, the cushioning effect of the elastic mouthguard material between the teeth can help to protect them as they smash against each other, relieve the stress to the jawjoints, and also reduces the overall concussion suffered by the brain. Sometimes a blow to the chin can cause the delicate jawjoint to fracture, but the impact force can be reduced by a mouthguard.

"THE WEARING OF MOUTHGUARDS TO PROTECT TEETH IS STRONGLY ADVISED DURING ALL CONTACT SPORTS."

Mouth accidents happen most commonly to young children between the ages of 6-11 as they often fall whilst playing.

Although it is not practical for children to be wearing mouthguards all the time, children who have remarkably projecting two front teeth which protrude (stick-out) too far forwards are often advised to have them retruded (moved back) early by orthodontic treatment so that in the event of an accident, the extent of damage suffered by these teeth is less serious.

FIRST-AID TREATMENT FOR A TOOTH KNOCKED OUT

A Baby Tooth:
1. Wash the wound with clean water.
2. Stop the bleeding with a moist hankerchief or cotton wool compressed against the cut lips for 5 minutes.
3. Stop the bleeding of the empty socket by biting or pressing a moist hankerchief or cotton wool directly onto it.
4. Without delay, rush your child to your dentist !

An Adult Tooth:
1. Pick up the tooth by the crown only, and never contaminate the root by touching it.
2. Rinse it briefly for 10 seconds under a cold running tap, just to flush off debris, and push it back into the socket. (never use soap, detergent, or any chemicals). Go straight to your dentist.
3. Alternatively put it in a glass of milk;or just in the mouth between the cheek and the teeth.
4. Call your dentist quickly and get there within 30 minutes if you wish to have that tooth back into the socket. Re-implanting the tooth back-in beyond 30 minutes may become less successful! (Never place a knocked-out baby tooth back into its socket, it will be rejected. Re-implantation only works with adult tooth, but even not always).

Treatment

After a front tooth is knocked, the criteria is the health of the nerve. If there is damage to the nerve it must be treated.

Whilst enamel and dentine fractures can be restored with fillings as usual, fractures beyond these, including the fracture of the jaws and jawjoints, are more complex. Tests for its vitality is done, but if the nerve dies, the tooth will turn grey as the tissues inside start to decompose and release by-products. A tooth slightly knocked may become loose and tender at first, but usually gains firmness after about 3 weeks.

If it had been displaced, it could be repositioned back to its original position by hand before it starts to heal. If the root is fractured, things become a bit more complicated. All decisions for treatment are decided as according to the actual condition.

X-ray images, vitality and mobility tests are conducted at regular intervals to monitor the progress.

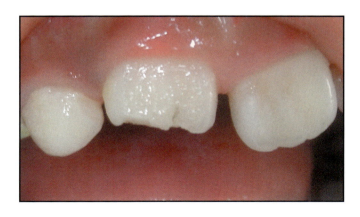

A Fractured Front Tooth

13. Old Fillings And Overhangs

"TEETH CAN BE TOTALLY DESTROYED BY LEAKING FILLINGS!"

Beware, the old ones tend to leak.

All restorations such as fillings, crowns and bridges should be checked regularly but especially the older ones which had been in your mouth for over a decade. Once your teeth are all patched up with fillings, there are more places for them to leak and cause decay inside. This is known as recurrent decay, or recurrent caries. Old amalgams and composite resin fillings are prone to leakages. They tend to deform or disintegrate over time, and amalgams can even break up into many multiple fragments.

For most of the tooth decay that are treated for adults, they are mostly recurrent as they always occur under the existing old fillings, crowns and bridges. Unlike children, it is less common to find fresh new cavities in the "virgin teeth" of adults.

This is perhaps the commonest cause for tooth extractions in adults, and the first to go is almost always those 1st molar teeth, those very first ones that had erupted at the age of 6 and were typically never protected with fissure sealants.

You won't even feel it. You'll even doubt it when your dentist tells you.

You may feel sensitivity or pain if the nerve is alive, but this is in fact good because it tells you to go to your dentist and get it fixed. However if the nerve is dead, you won't feel anything while things continually leak in. Eventually the whole tooth inside becomes rotten whilst you are completely unaware, until it is too late. Teeth are commonly extracted as a result of this. There may not be any pain throughout the process if the nerve dies slowly, or if the tooth had already been root-filled. The insensitive root-filling material is simply dissolved by the influx of contaminated salivary fluids and it rots inside with the rest of the tooth. Leakages are never obvious, for most of the time, the filling stays in and everything feels normal. However, when the filling finally falls out, it does so only because it has become completely embedded in decay all around and can no longer be retained. Recurrent decay is another major cause for a tooth extraction and is caused by the failure of old fillings, crowns and bridges to maintain their water-tight seal for the tooth, over time. The fact that these crowns or fillings still feel intact serves only to give you a false sense of security. When it is discovered too late, the only option left is an extraction! This happens all too often. The thing you should know is that rotten teeth which had been root-filled and restored with huge old fillings, crowns or post-crowns are very brittle and are indeed very difficult to extract in one piece. They are ready to crumble into many fragments the moment the extraction forceps squeeze on these for a good grip. In many instances the crumbling tooth needs to be dissected out fragment by fragment by means of a minor surgery.

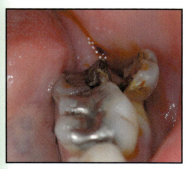

Recurrent decay occurred extensively inside, around the old metal filling. The weakened tooth fractured and it was extracted.

Abundance of plaque in the mouth due to poor oral hygiene is commonly blamed, causing decay around old fillings.

Whereas small fillings at the front and top surfaces of teeth are easily cleaned, fillings which extend between back teeth are unreachable to the toothbrush, and are often never flossed. As a result, this is the most common site for recurrent decay.

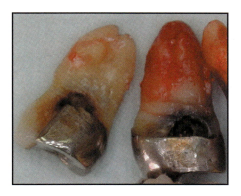

DECAY OCCURS BETWEEN, AROUND AND UNDERNEATH OLD FILLINGS, UNSUSPECTINGLY. BEWARE !

Fillings, crowns and bridges are all equally prone to leakages over time. These must always be discovered as early as possible by your dentist at regular dental check-ups, and images from the x-rays are particularly useful for detecting these.

OVERHANGS.

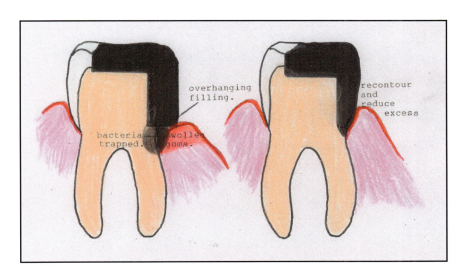

The most destructive fillings, crowns or bridges are those which are too bulbous and have ledges which overhang at the gums.

They trap a lot of food and bacteria which is not only uncomfortable for you, and quite impossible to clean well, but they are very harmful; initiating decay to the tooth and destroying the gums too. If you should floss at these and the floss catches and shreds, you have just detected the overhangs by yourself. You must request your dentist to have them all either reshaped, or replaced. Every dentist immediately recognizes the significance of overhangs through training, so never hesitate to highlight them at your next visit. There are actually special kits for correcting overhangs in every dental clinic. The destruction over time caused by overhangs can lead to early tooth losses, and this is totally preventable.

14. Missing Teeth

The consequences of tooth losses are obvious; eating, speaking, smiling and singing are all affected, but without many of them in the mouth, the jaws do not have enough teeth to rest on and the biting is disturbed. This will cause pain to the jawjoints and great discomforts to the jaw muscles. The remainder of the teeth must bear all the forces of biting, overstressing them.

Losing all back teeth could result in great stresses on the fronts, wearing them quickly and leading to their early losses.

Our teeth all function together in balance with each other, and if extracted, they should be replaced as soon as possible.

The Consequences Of A Tooth Loss.
Losing adult teeth usually starts with the 1st adult molar, as a consequence of tooth decay. Fissure sealants help to prevent it.

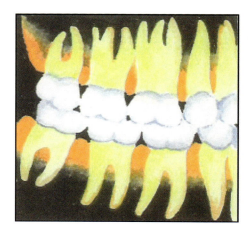 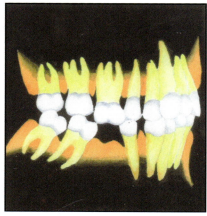

Before An Extraction　　After An Extraction

1. The unopposed upper tooth will come down towards the space.
2. The teeth on either side of the space will tilt at an angle towards the space.
3. Small gaps are created between the teeth which had moved.

This collapse seriously compromises the effectiveness of chewing on that whole side of the mouth.

This is very common and it is a good example to show how the loss of one tooth can affect the rest of the teeth.

The Loss Of A Front Tooth.

The commonest reason for people to lose their front tooth is because of previous mouth injuries, whether they were struck by an object, had a sports injury, or an accidental fall. Children are generally more prone to these sorts of injuries than adults. They are simply more accident-prone due to their activeness and their undeveloped coordination. Contact sports contribute greatly to the loss of front teeth and players wear mouthguards nowadays during play. This standard equipment had saved many people's front teeth.

Leaking post-crowns of front teeth is another common cause as it can allow bacteria to enter and contaminate the remainder of the root. The decay inside the root becomes so extensive that it is subsequently extracted.

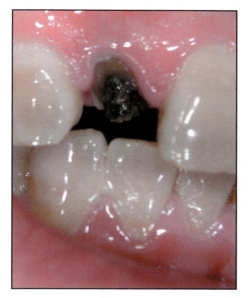 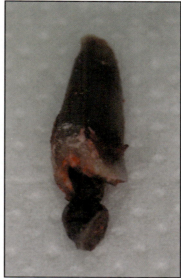

There are various ways for replacing teeth and in recent years dental technology had advanced considerably in this area.

Immediate Front Tooth Replacement.

Dental Implants.

Dental implants have become very popular and can nowadays be used to immediately replace a very broken front tooth.

You can literally have the front tooth extracted and the dental implant inserted back in within the hour simply under a local anaesthetic. Dental implants are getting better and better as we speak and nowadays they can be gently inserted right into the empty socket after the tooth is extracted. Only the tip of the implant is frictionally engaged with the bone for an initial stability as new bone forms around the implant. As the socket heals, the bone heals naturally around onto the dental implant surface and there is never the need for "tight-screwing" of the implant during its insertion. This is why it is virtually painless, ideal, and highly successful. This is known as an "Immediate Dental Implant" and the criteria for this is the total absence of infection and pus inside the socket where the dental implant is to be inserted.

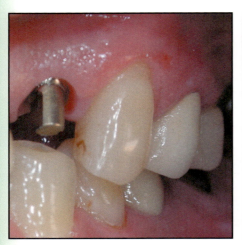 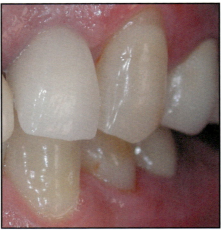 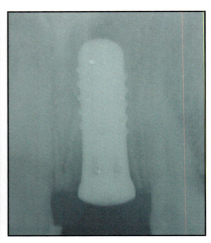

Dental implants are suitable for adults, but not for children as their jaws and teeth are still growing. For them, a temporary denture could be provided in the meantime until their jawgrowths had finalized.

Bridges.

If you should decide to have a bridge constructed to replace your missing front tooth, you should wait for 2 months after the extraction because the bone around the socket shrinks considerably afterwards. It tends to shrink 2-3 mm in the first 2 months but stabilizes afterwards. If the bridge is made promptly after the extraction, you might find a 2-3 mm space developing underneath it 2 months later, and this gap is very noticeable.

Thinking Of Teeth Replacements?

Well here are the 3 main choices:
1. Removable dentures
2. Fixed dental bridges.
3. Dental implants.

1. Dentures.

Dentures, or removable false teeth, are the historical method for replacing teeth and remains the simplest and cheapest to date. When there is enough healthy teeth remaining, a removable partial denture supported by natural teeth may be considered and these have metal hooks to engage around the remaining teeth which provide their stability. If too many teeth are missing, the denture is seated only on the gums and is less stable. This causes discomforts and soreness during chewing and talking as it shifts, rubs and scratches the gums. It takes time to adapt to them. The denture base itself is made usually of plastic, except for the metal hooks, known as clasps, which wrap around the remaining teeth. The teeth are also usually made of plastic. A few visits are needed to make the denture. Dentures can be made entirely of acrylic (plastic) or with a Cobalt-chromium metal base for added strength, but the latter is slightly more costly. In general if you have to wear dentures, it's always best to go for the cobalt-chromium metal based ones.

Missing Teeth

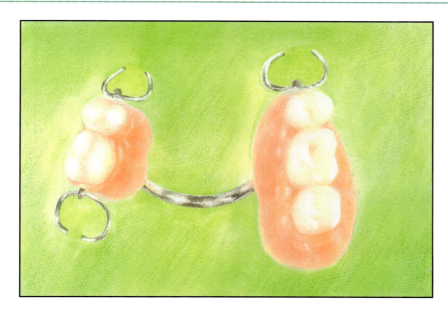

Impressions of your mouth are taken and sent to the dental laboratory for construction. Wax-bite records are taken at a second visit to determine the height, desired positions and proper colour of your new teeth. The dentures are then made and are next fitted in the mouth at the third appointment but follow-up visits are needed for adjusting them properly in the mouth. Dentures always feel rather awkward and their chewing forces are far weaker in comparison to natural teeth.

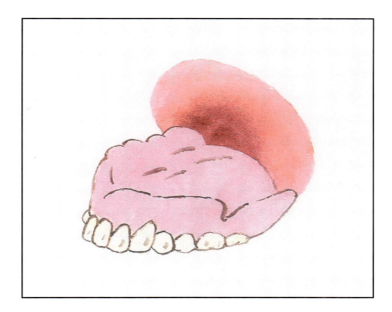

When you have completely no teeth, a complete denture is simply "seated" on the gums. Dentures occupy the larger areas in the mouth to distribute the chewing forces, so it might cause you gaggings. Some people adapt to wearing dentures better than others, but if you've lost all your teeth and don't have enough bone for dental implants, dentures are your best bet .

Dentures must never be worn during sleeping. They must be brushed and kept cleaned, kept soaked in water preferably with a cleanser whilst they are not in the mouth. Any remaining teeth must be brushed and flossed in the usual way.

Disadvantages Of Dentures.

Dentures are less stable during chewing, talking, or singing and their biting forces are weaker. Any metal hooks will collect food and bacteria around the remaining teeth which can damage them. If badly designed, they can put incorrect pressure on the natural teeth causing them to tip, and if these already have gum disease, wearing badly-fitting dentures can lead to more tooth-losses. Their metal clasps can cause decay to occur around the remaining teeth they hook around, leading to toothache.

As the bone underneath continues to shrink, the denture becomes looser over time, and would require repeated replacements, or adding more plastic layers on them known as relines, to compensate for it. Heavy biting forces on the gums may increase the rate and extent of the bone shrinking underneath, rather like skis on snow, especially if it is the gum-borne lower denture. This is why dentures should try to cover as huge an area of the mouth as you can possibly tolerate to spread the load and reduce the shrinkage of the bone underneath. The plastic teeth can scratch, crack and stain, over time.

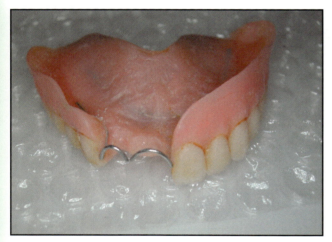 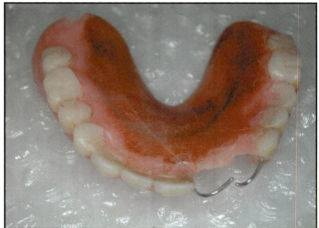

2. Fixed Bridges.

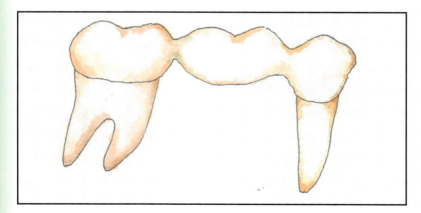 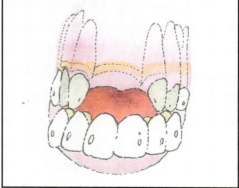

Fixed bridges have become popular in preference to wearing dentures because they can be permanently fixed to the natural teeth which are healthy and strong. They are considered permanent and do not lose stability even when the bone underneath shrinks. They provide comfort, good stability, aesthetics and sufficient strength for chewing. They do not have the huge plastic bases and flanges as in dentures and feel slim in the mouth. However, dental bridges are more expensive than dentures and require the healthy teeth on either side of the gap to be filed down for support, imposing extra burden on them.

A fixed bridge consists of the pontic teeth (the artificial tooth replacing the missing ones) which are splinted with crowns on either side in one single casting and is cemented permanently onto the natural teeth on either side of the gap. It is important that the existing teeth are strong and healthy enough to provide the support needed. Teeth already with gum disease could be destroyed quicker if they are used for supporting a bridge.

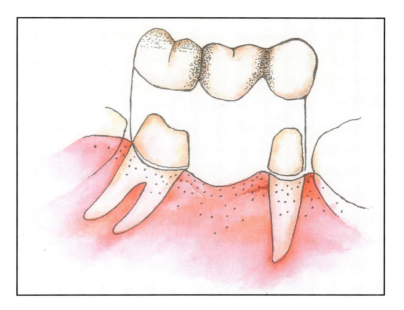

The advantage of a fixed bridge is that you can talk and eat without worrying about it moving. The only drawback with bridges is that they do require teeth on either side of the gap to be drastically filed down even if they are completely healthy and free of fillings. In a sense, they are innocently sacrificed for the bridge. (On the other hand, it's more acceptable if they already needed to be crowned).

A mold is subsequently taken and sent for bridge construction at the dental laboratory. The bridge is subsequently cemented permanently by your dentist. A bridge is made of a metal framework, alone (a gold alloy, or other metal alloy), or plus a superficial layer of porcelain for aesthetics. Porcelain alone is prone to fracturing and a metal framework is always needed for strength. The question is whether you need porcelain added on it for aesthetics, because they bear the risk of fracturing.

Fixed bridges require extra meticulous brushing as they trap food and plaque underneath. Cleaning and flossing underneath the bridge requires dedication to maintain the health of the natural teeth within, which are providing their support.

The disadvantage of bridges is that should anything go wrong with an individual tooth supporting it, if there should be decay or leakages, the whole bridge has to be replaced.

3. Dental Implants

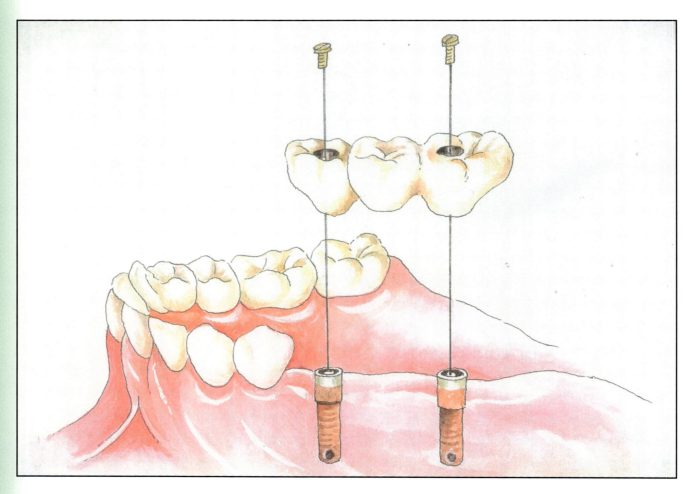

    A dental implant is an artificial tooth root replacement and is based on the discovery by Professor Per-Ingvar Branemark that titanium could be successfully incorporated into bone when bone cells grow onto the surface of the implanted titanium. This forms a structural and functional connection between the living bone and the implant. This is revolutionary because for the first time, the roots of the extracted teeth can be replaced. A dental implant is inserted into the jawbone. The bone remodels around the dental implant as it would around natural tooth roots. The success rate is about 95% overall, and it has become a very reliable and successful procedure. A dental implant is a biocompatible screw-like fixture, typically made of 99.75 pure titanium. The threading mainly serves to engage the dental implant to the bone for an initial stability, but after 3 months, the bone integrates with the surface of the titanium for a tight fusion. This is known as osseointegration. Once it has fused to the jawbone, virtually anything can be connected onto it. Dental implants are basically pillars anchored into the jawbone to provide its independent support for all artificial teeth selectable to be mounted onto them; be it a single crown, one end of a bridge or an over-denture. In theory there are no upper age limits for dental implants so long as one is in good general health. (Smoking, however, can reduce the success rate by about 5%).

Titanium

Body reactions or allergies to titanium does not occur as humans naturally ingest a large amount of titanium in many chemical forms as part of the daily diet. About 40% of the total amount taken into the body, or about 30 micrograms are metabolized each day. This is approximately 10,000 times the amount of titanium potentially delivered by a dental implant existing in a jawbone. Titanium is considered safe and inert in the body. The dental implant in your mouth would not set off the alarm at airport security checks, and you won't need to have them removed for a **MRI** scan at the hospital.

The Procedure. - For A Single Dental Implant

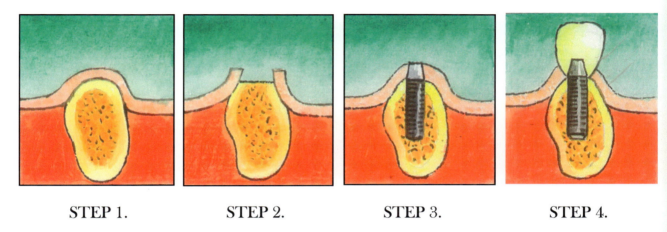

STEP 1.   STEP 2.   STEP 3.   STEP 4.

STEP 1. With the use of an x-ray or a CT scan, the height and thickness of the bone of the missing tooth is measured.

STEP 2. A thin cut on the gum is done to expose the bone underneath and it is drilled to form a socket for the Dental Implant.

STEP 3. A carefully chosen suitable Dental Implant is inserted into the socket of the bone, and the gum is stitched back.

STEP 4. After 3 months, the titanium is fused to the bone (osseointegration); a tooth is directly screwed onto the Dental Implant.

The insertion procedure actually takes less than an hour, including administering a local anaesthetic, and the 1 or 2 tiny stitches.

There is usually very little bleeding because the anaesthetic itself constricts all the capillaries, effectively limiting the blood flow.

Surprisingly there is also rarely any bleeding, swelling and pain afterwards. Pain occurs only if an infection develops, commonly due to poor oral hygiene, smoking, or the wearing of infected old dentures over it.

Dental Implant Bridge

Dental implants have been proven to be so successful that nowadays they can be surgically placed and fitted with the crown immediately under certain ideal conditions. Dental implants are not affected by tooth decay, but they could be affected by gum infections. Bacteria can still leak in via the gums to contaminate the surfaces of the dental implant, causing it to fail.

Meticulous brushing at the dental implants remains critical for their longterm survival. Dental implants does provide the ultimate solution to tooth loss, and can provide the enormous forces needed for chewing. They are titanium roots in jaws which can provide rigidity and stability for the crowns or bridges screwed onto them, giving you back your beautiful smile. You can certainly bite an apple with them.

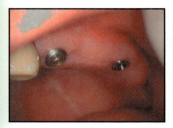 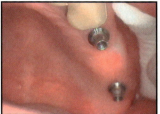 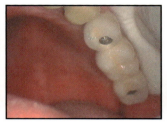 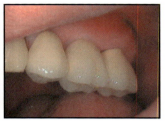

Dental implants can last for decades and once they have osseointegrated successfully and are well cared for, they have almost no time limits. Repeated replacements of the crown or bridge on them are rarely necessary. However, if needed, the old ones can simply be unscrewed out and the new ones screwed on, and all done within minutes. Alternatively the same bridge can be unscrewed, have the worn porcelain completely resurfaced for a fractional cost, be screwed on again, and it's as good as new. The first dental implant was placed in 1965 and it still remains in good function today, but the dental implants of today are even better ! Previously people had to wait for 6 months for the bone to grow around them, but the newest ones can become just as strong in 3 weeks ! In some cases you could have all the implants and the teeth in the mouth in one day. This is the "Same Day Teeth" technique.

The only dangers for dental implants are bruxism (night-grinding), heavy smoking and poor oral hygiene.

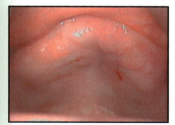 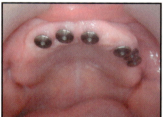 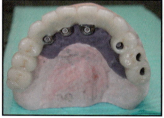 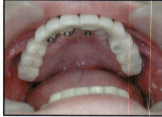

Are Dental Implants Suitable For You?

This must be discussed with your dentist as it does depend on your health condition and the available amount of bone in your jaws. Only your dentist can evaluate the answer for you depending on your particular situation. It is also important to discuss any risks involved, and the cost of treatment. They are however far more expensive than dentures and bridges because they include the replacement of the tooth roots in addition to the tooth crowns. However, they can provide enormous forces for chewing superseding the natural teeth as they are absolutely rigid within the jawbone. Dental implants are potentially lifetime investments.

Dental implants replicate well the missing natural tooth roots and they allow bone to continue remodeling around them throughout life. This preserves the dimensional integrity of your jaw skeleton and maintains your youthful face appearance. The ability to preserve youth is the true feature provided exclusively by dental implants when you have lost most or all of your teeth.

15. Cosmetic dentistry

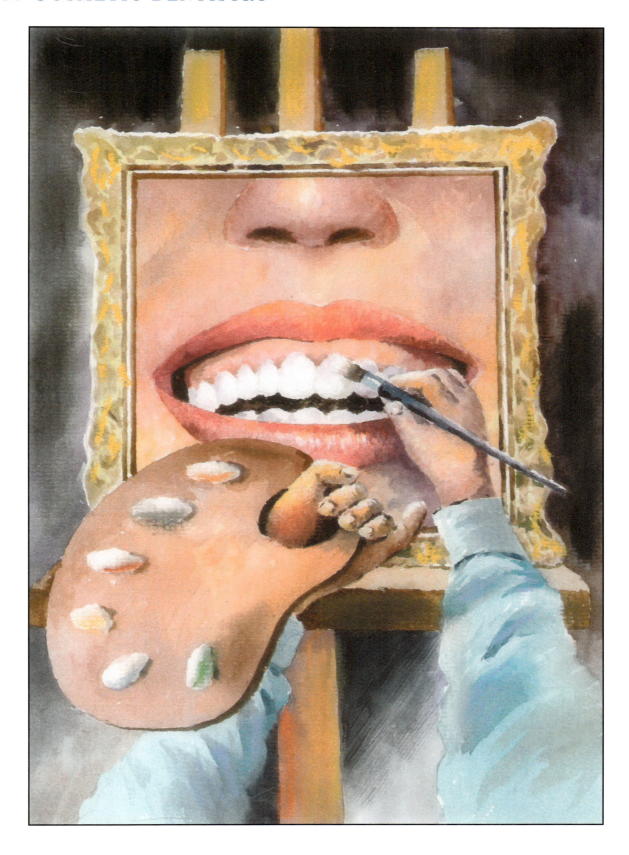

Cosmetic dentistry is not necessarily a frivolous self-indulgence in vanity as many people perceive it to be. Health is beauty.

In the past, dental treatment was primarily focused on the repairing of damages to teeth by decay, extraction of teeth due to decay and gum disease, and missing teeth were replaced by removable dentures. Only the very wealthy, or those who had depended on their smile to make their living, such as Hollywood stars or famous people, would take seriously the steps to improve their smile. Nowadays, cosmetic dentistry has become very popular as people are becoming more aware about their appearances. Speech is affected by the teeth rotated or being out of line. An adolescent's self-esteem is most vulnerable to the negative opinions of his classmates and adults who have never had their crooked teeth corrected soon realize their awkward appearances as they smile to their colleagues. Business careers could sometimes be affected by unfavourable first impressions. Many options have nowadays become available at affordable costs. Improving your smile with cosmetic treatments involves improving the state of the teeth and gums. Teeth positions in the mouth, their proportional shape and form, their colour, surface texture and lifelike translucencies are all of concern.

"YOUR FRIENDLY SMILE CAN OPEN DOORS FOR YOU".

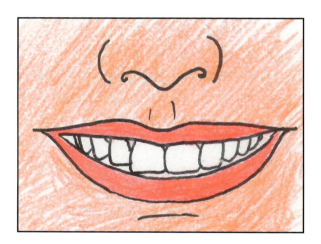

"The shadow of your smile. . . . . "

First Impressions

First impressions are very critical and always have lasting effects. The most successful people of today take this fact very seriously . They spend time to take meticulous care of their faces, their hair, their fingernails, make-up, dresswear and they would always check themselves in front of the mirror whenever they walked past one. A smile is often the first thing we do when we meet people, and it is the most friendly gesture expressed so well by our body language that it is done conveniently without words. A smile which shows an unhygienic mouth with tobacco-stained or decayed teeth would demolish the general attraction of a person. It's like wearing a neat suit for a business occasion but shaking hands with grit underneath the finger nails and dandruff scattered on the shoulders. Although crooked teeth can be acceptable and is often forgiven, poor personal hygiene isn't and is reflective of a person. Having bad breath at the same time would further discredit one's attention to hygiene and this can adversely affect one's image. When we flash our teeth, we would leave an impression, albeit good or bad. Hollywood stars can make such impacts whenever they flash their teeth in front of the camera, or on posters. Their graceful images heavily depend on their good teeth conditions. Flashing a smile with straight and healthy teeth is one feature equally attainable by all and serves as one's social weapon of charm. Although the rest of us are not celebrities, it is equally worth the costs and efforts to correct our teeth as we too have our own images to live up to in our own social circles. The enthusiasm associated with seeking cosmetic treatments for teeth can often in essence improve their health and this is by far the most important by-product of the whole exercise. The costs could be limited to only improving dental health, and for the blessed people who had their teeth maintained perfectly from birth, they already have the perfect smile. Whilst it is unfortunate that teeth lack the ability to regenerate throughout life, unlike our skin, nails and hair, the fortunate thing is that the smile does not change. This feature is an advantage for teeth because if well-cared for and apart from some wear and tear, teeth can remain largely unaffected by age. Whilst the rest of the body deteriorates as skin wrinkles appear and the hair turns white, the perfect smile can faithfully remain unaltered to the grave.

The perfect smile boosts self-esteem, and the million dollar smile could get you anywhere! People who tend to smile readily are generally more impacting and are successful in all personal, social and business aspects. They feel enough confidence to charm people every time and they know it too. They could also know how to gain better attention during all social and business meetings. Self-confidence is in itself attractive. In life, feeling good about ourselves is almost everything. In contrast, feeling inadequate or insecure is mentally destructive. It's nice to have something about our faces that we could be proud enough to show.

Everything we do in life is influenced by our minds, and our attitudes towards problems are mostly determined by our mental states. Positive thinking is the most vital ingredient we need to adopt in order to survive the stresses and burdens we face in life.

There are few guidelines for combating stress and depression because it is primarily to do with our own minds that few others could truly comprehend. Although having good rest, nutrition, daily exercise, reading a book and so on do have their benefits, a healthy body, however, can lead to a healthy mind. Having the perfect teeth could positively boost a person's self-esteem, and if the sense of feeling great could encourage more smiling and laughing, it adds a positive cheer to life.

"A BEAUTIFUL RADIANT SMILE IS ONE OF THE GREATEST ASSETS ANY PERSON CAN HAVE"

Children and teenagers are especially affected by the imperfect appearances of their teeth especially if they are discoloured, very crooked, abnormal or missing. They make a conscious effort to avoid smiling, trying to cover-up their teeth everytime.

They are most affected when they are openly teased at school about their unattractive teeth and those with very crooked teeth are particularly noticed. Their confidence and social performances reach an all time low until their smile is restored.

The effects on any person having their smile restored are most dramatic, almost like bringing them back to life ! They smile more, talk more, sing more, dominate parties with their presence, and are openly more cheerful afterwards. The correction of a smile is one of the most appreciated and gratifying services a dentist can render to a patient and the orthodontic straightening of crooked teeth for children, teenagers and adults forms an imperative first step towards the perfect smile.

So What Is The Perfect Smile?

Well at least one could imagine that all the teeth are healthy, they are perfectly straight, have no gaps between them, and appear complete in a smile. The smile looks very attractive with whiter teeth because it is associated with youth and vitality. Those front teeth, in particular, could mark the feature of a person's face because they are most impressionable. Before teeth can look perfect, they do need to be normal in their shapes and sizes. The teeth must meet together nicely as they bite together, and the smile looks symmetrical and comfortable. The gums must also look pink and healthy without signs of disease, scalloping neatly around all the necks of the teeth. The proportion of gums and teeth must be reasonably balanced, otherwise the excess mass of fleshy gums overlapping a set of very short and small teeth makes the smile look very gummy.

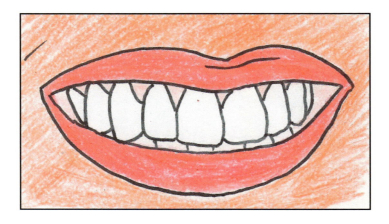

The Aesthetic Zone.

If you think about it, you will realize that your mouth and your jaws form approximately one-third of your face, and if you excluded the forehead, it actually makes up half of your face. Your mouth is always the focus of attention whenever you speak.

Women wear lipsticks to highlight their attractive mouths, and as they flash their teeth with talking or smiling, you will glimpse their conditions. Those upper front teeth would always leave an impression. All those teeth displayed in a smile are said to be in the aesthetic zone, or appearance zone, and mainly include 6-10 of the upper teeth across the mouth from lip corner to lip corner, and a few of the lower front teeth. Cosmetic dentistry is concerned with the teeth appearances in this zone.

The Aesthetic Zone.

The number of teeth readily displayed varies from person to person depending on the size and shape of their mouths as the lips extend, and the degree of muscular stretch of the lips varies from person to person. It is those teeth displayed in the smile that has by far the most important effect on your appearance and they form the basis for cosmetic dentistry. When most people smile, they typically display the four upper front teeth, the upper canines and the upper premolars on both sides of the mouth. If you ever wish to whiten your teeth in a smile, whether by tooth bleaching, or with porcelain crowns or veneers, these must be included in the treatment so that they can all be done together at the same time.

The beauty of a person's face is heavily determined by its symmetry and proportionality, and a symmetrical smile produced by the symmetrical positioning of all teeth and centered within your face is most critical. Wearing braces will do this for you.

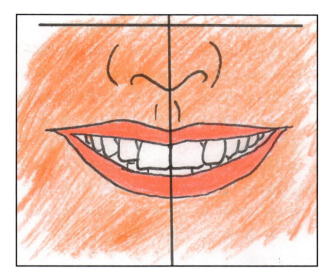 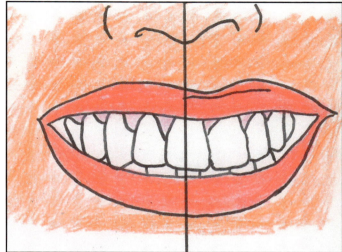

SYMMETRICAL SMILE   ASYMMETRICAL SMILE

You can check this by yourself with a self-portrait photograph, drawing a vertical line down the midline of your face.

If the line passes down between your two upper front teeth (Central Incisors), then your smile is symmetrical. Your smile should also be balanced being leveled with your eyes, and that your smile is not somewhat slanting at an angle.

YOUR FACIAL SKELETON.

If your face is not straight because your jaws are not balanced, the only way to improve them would have to be to correct them with surgery. Correcting jawbones in this way is known as orthognathic surgery and is performed by the specialist Oral Surgeons. In the meantime the teeth are also corrected with orthodontic treatment in order for you to bite correctly after the jaws have been repositioned correctly. Oral surgeons and orthodontists work hand in hand during the whole process. The improvements are often so gratifying and dramatic that they are always worth doing. Correcting the jaws using surgery may sound too extreme, but they are meant to make extreme improvements! Surprisingly they take only a couple of hours to complete, a week for recovery, and 3 months for complete bone healing, with thanks to the advancement of technology in this field. People who have done it are always a whole lot better off and far happier than having to live the rest of their lives with their distorted jaws ! You almost couldn't recognize them afterwards. It's like a different life for them and the happiness within them after being released from their complex is astounding. Their social activities begin to flourish!

Things You Should Know About Teeth

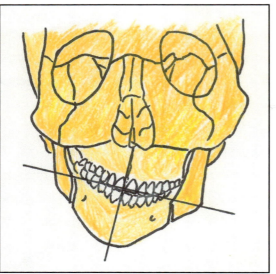 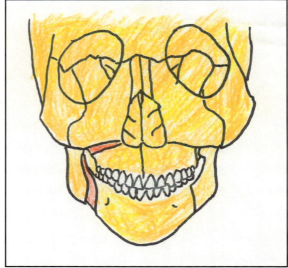

A slanting smile could be improved by horizontally straightening the jaws.

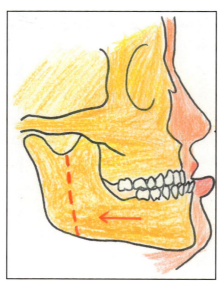 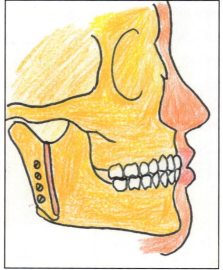

A protruding lower jaw could be moved back to become balanced with the upper jaw.

There are literally millions of people today who have very protruding lower jaws, and whilst a mild protrusion may appear masculine for men, it might not appear quite so attractive for women. The bite is almost certainly completely wrong, but many hesitate at the thought of surgery. This jaw feature is so common that if you look around at the bus-stop, or on the train, you will almost certainly spot at least one person with it. Jaw correction is as important as the need for orthodontics.

A Good Foundation.

Wearing braces, and/or correcting jaws, is by far the most effective way to achieve the best foundation for the perfect smile.

The beauty of your smile is heavily influenced by the straightness of your jaws and teeth. This leaves the colour of the teeth, the quality and colour of the artificial materials they are restored with, and also the health of teeth and gums to enhance the smile. The perfect smile must never contain stains, nor any signs of disease; the teeth must appear healthy, normal and natural.

16. Positioning Teeth

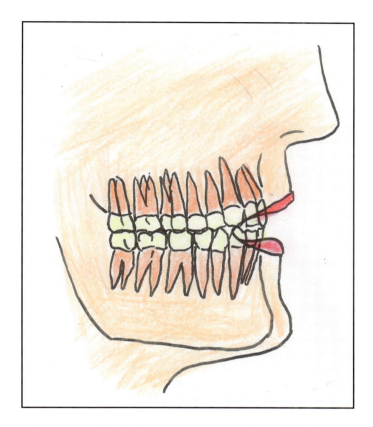

    The positioning of your smile is important, starting with the straight setting of all your teeth. Your smile will look best when positioned leveled and centered on your face with the teeth all angled correctly behind your lips and cheeks. This also requires the roots of teeth to become correctly positioned within the jawbones, and that the upper and lower jaws have grown in balance with each other. The front teeth can have a profound influence on the profile of the lips, which in itself is a major facial feature. The field of orthodontics is primarily concerned with all of these factors and their treatments would provide the best foundation for the perfect smile. The correction of overjets, overbites, cross bites, deep bites, open bites, midline shifts and gaps between teeth are all part of this tedious and lengthy treatment which not only aim for the best positions of teeth to bite together comfortably, but will provide lifelong good appearances for your smile.

What Is An Overjet?

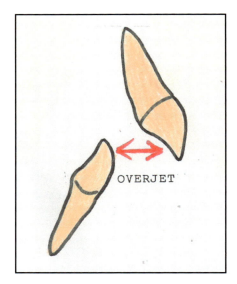

This is defined as the horizontal overlap of the incisor teeth.

The protruding front teeth can have dramatic effects on your lip profile, but in the event of an accident, as in a trauma to the face, these front teeth and lips would be seriously injured. "Goofy teeth" must ideally be corrected before they get knocked!

What Is An Overbite?

This is defined as the vertical overlap of the front teeth.
When the upper front teeth completely overlaps the lower, this is a deep bite.
If there is no overlap at all, with a space between the front teeth, this is an open bite

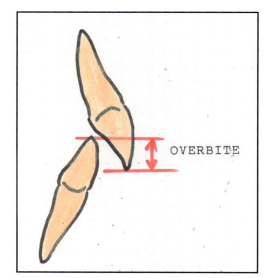

A deep overbite: people who have deep overbites have shorter faces than they deserve, but with correction, the face height increases back to normal.

76

WHAT IS A CROSSBITE?

A crossbite is a transverse discrepancy in the arch relationship, or the reversed position of one or more teeth. The tooth is said to be in an instanding position to the bite and commonly collects stains and dental plaque on and around it.

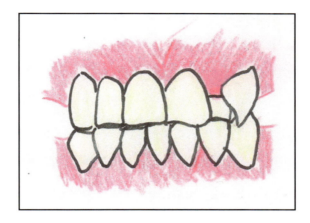

All the crookedness, gaps and bad positionings of teeth are corrected by orthodontic treatments and the best time for this is during childhood, starting at around the age of 11-13 yrs. old after the baby teeth have all shed. Teeth are commonly crowded and some may need to be extracted in order for the rest to become straight. Soon after the chosen teeth have been extracted, the brackets can be bonded onto the teeth for wires to be fitted. The whole process for all the teeth to be straightened may take 18 months or more, depending on the situation, and the wires need to be changed regularly monthly or bi-monthly. The reason why it takes so long is because the teeth cannot be moved too quickly using too heavy forces otherwise it would be too painful.

Teeth move as a result of a low but continuous and persuasive force applied to them when the discomfort caused is minimal.

In general teeth should not be exerted to move more than 1mm per month.

There is no true upper age limit for considering orthodontics although it is preferably done during the growing ages. At school, children are used to seeing braces but once they start working, they could feel too embarrassed to wear them. The correction of incorrect bites can make great improvements towards the comfort of the jaws in function and one's general appearance.

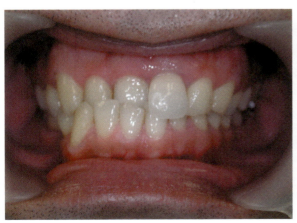
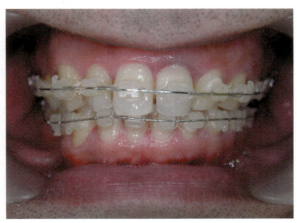

For Adults.

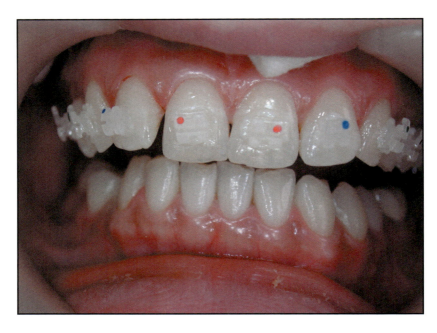

White Ceramic Brackets (The Colour Labels Peel Off).

Nowadays, the availability of white ceramic brackets has become popular for the adult patient and they work equally well for handling the very crooked cases. They look far better than the metal brackets and have encouraged many adults to straighten their crooked teeth. Lingual brackets, or brackets placed behind the teeth have also found their fans, but the process is far more tedious and can cost considerably more. The introduction of the invisible braces has given hope for some adults, using a sequence of custom-made transparent mouthguards, but they work very well in certain cases. The case selection is very critical for these to work effectively, and target those cases with mildly crooked problems. The teeth are marginally shaved at their sides to narrow them down in order to provide extra space. This way teeth do not need to be extracted for it. A series of custom-made clear and invisible aligners are provided, each worn for two weeks and changed in sequence. The results for selected cases are quite astounding. There are no brackets and wires and the clear plastic aligners tightly fitting onto the teeth creates tensional forces which persuades their movements. However, they cannot as yet handle the "very crooked cases" requiring extreme and drastic movements of teeth as compared with the certainties and capabilities offered by the traditional devices of metal or ceramic brackets, wires and elastics. Quite often these invisible braces need to be finished in the traditional way, and thus the good old conventional brackets, wires and elastics are once again employed in the final stages to "finish the rest of the job".

17. Whitening Teeth

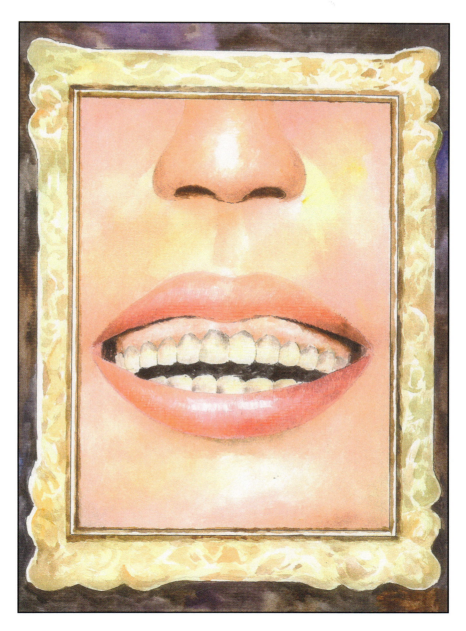

Yellow Teeth Is Common.
Now don't we all wished we had white teeth ? We actually did when we were young, but as we got older, they got yellower.

By the time we reach old age, they're almost brown. The degree of tooth discolouration varies a lot from person to person, from the slight yellowing in most to the grossly dark and heavily stained type in some. Sometimes there are patterns of grey bands running across each tooth, with pittings and irregular surface texture. Discoloured teeth can have much the same effect on self-esteem and confidence as having no teeth at all. Some people hide their teeth all the time simply because of their discolouration.

Discoloured Teeth

We always assume that everyone has healthy and straightened white teeth because anything different would look abnormal. Although teeth are most attractive when they are dazzling with whiteness, and look sensual for women wearing red lipsticks, human teeth are never naturally quite so dazzling. Newly erupted teeth during childhood may be very white to start with, when the enamel is thickest, but as enamel wears with age (through daily brushing, acid drinks, abrasive foods) the teeth just turn yellow. Increase of enamel wear allows the dentine inside to become more apparent, and as we all know, dentine is yellow.

The harder we brush, the yellower the teeth gets and this is a common mistake. If you wish to whiten your teeth safely and effectively, tooth bleaching may be your best solution, and this has become very successful and popular in recent years.

There are two basic types of discolourations, or stainings caused to teeth; the first and most common is known as the extrinsic staining which can be readily removed by professional cleaning. the second is known as the intrinsic staining which cannot readily be removed effectively and is by far the more difficult to tackle. People who have very dark teeth have been constantly aware of them since childhood.

Extrinsic Staining.

Extrinsic staining is the staining of teeth is the removable stains on the outer surfaces of teeth which are caused by foods which stain. Coffee, tea, tobacco, red wine, can all effect staining to teeth and these can all be removed by a visit to the dentist.

Some mouthwashes which contain chlorhexidine gluconate can stain all the teeth if with prolonged usage, but they too can be removed professionally. Many toothpastes nowadays contain ingredients which can help to remove some tooth stains. Heavy scrubbing with your toothbrush in a massive attempt to remove all of your tooth stains can be very abrasive for your teeth. Everyone will collect extrinsic staining from time to time, and regular visits to your dentist will remove all those stains for you safely, quickly and effectively. Tooth polishing removes all the food-stains from your teeth and is the simplest and fastest way to restore your beautiful smile.

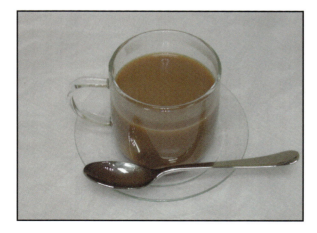
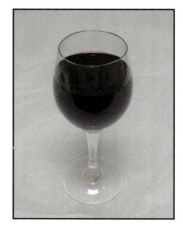

Beverages.   **Red wine.**

Intrinsic Staining.
Yellow Teeth

Intrinsic staining is the stained colour of the teeth after they were formed and they cannot be removed by simple cleaning.

In general, the colour of teeth is the same for all race and gender, but differs with age as they tend to yellow with time.

Decades of toothbrushing causes some wear to the enamel which allows the underlying yellow dentine to become apparent. The yellowing effect also depends on the actual colour density of the dentine. Another reason for teeth yellowing with age is because over time, the permeability of the teeth allows slow infusion of organic pigments from our chromogenic foods, like gravy and curry. However, tooth bleaching techniques can help to lighten the colour of yellowed teeth caused by such accumulation of food colour infusions and helps to rejuvenate them. Another reason for an odd tooth to appear dark is because it has a decomposing dead nerve inside. This could be caused by decay, or bacteria had leaked underneath the filling.

Cracked teeth can also allow passage of bacteria into the nerve and cause its decomposing, in which case if allowed to remain inside for too long, the by-products would stain the tooth structure heavily. To reverse this, the dead nerves are removed by root canal treatment, and the tooth can be bleached inside (also known as internal bleaching) to refreshen its colour, followed by placement of a beautiful porcelain jacket crown.

Tooth Whitening-(Tooth Bleaching).

Bleaching is the simplest, safest and most conservative way to whiten the teeth. It is done by means of exposing teeth to carbamide peroxide or hydrogen peroxide, which are oxidizing agents. It is nothing new and teeth have been bleached for many centuries without causing harm. The first bleaching of teeth was reported in 1848 when it was used for internal bleaching for (non-vital) dead teeth stained by decomposing dead nerve tissues. In-office bleaching of (vital) teeth with healthy nerves, was reportedly done in 1868, or 20 years later. In the early 1900's the in-office bleaching for vital teeth had evolved to include the use of heat and light to activate the bleaching process. However, although bleaching mouthwashes were available for the public did exist as early as 1893 using a 3% ether-peroxide mouthwash, the "dentist-prescribed-home-bleaching-kit" wearing a mouthguard with gel inside, at home, started in 1968. These bleaching techniques use some form of hydrogen peroxide in different concentrations and the mechanism of action appears to be the oxidation of organic pigments. Although the chemistry is not very well understood the bleaching works well, is harmless and results have an approximate lifespan of 1-3 years to life. The whitening results can be rather dramatic for the yellow discoloured teeth, lightening them up a few shades immediately, but this is not so effective for the very darkly stained teeth. Bleaching may certainly lighten the colour of the tooth, but it cannot correct any irregular surface colour patterns, texture, bandings, pittings which can sometimes be improved by special polishing techniques such as microabrasion and macroabrasion, done by the dentist.

Prior to dental bleaching, a good cleaning is best done to remove the extrinsic stains caused by tea, coffee, tobacco, and so on.

There are basically 2 ways of bleaching, depending on the concentrations of the peroxides, and the use of a light source.

1. **HOME BLEACHING.**
These can be purchased over-the-counter in the form of gels, and are placed in a mouthguard to be exposed on the teeth overnight, typically recommended for 1 to 2 weeks. However, results are slow, and the whitening may not be obvious. The same goes for the whitening tooth pastes, or whitening strips as they contain relatively low concentrations of peroxides and they are not used in conjunction with a light source. However, with relentless persistence, some marginal results are visible.

2. **60 MINUTES: IN-OFFICE POWER BLEACHING.**
This uses the higher concentration form of hydrogen peroxide, typically 35%, plus the use of a direct high intensity light source to trigger the bleaching reaction on the teeth. The teeth are firstly thoroughly cleaned, then they are isolated by a piece of rubber-dam, to protect the gums and mouth from the gel. The gel is then coated onto all of the tooth front surfaces, which will be exposed to the high intensity light for 5-7 minutes. The gel is now rubbed off the teeth, followed by a second new coating of gel. This process is then repeated for 6 times. The gel is then washed off completely, and a fluoride gel is applied to the teeth for 1 minute, to replenish the surface layer with fluoride ions.

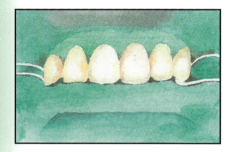 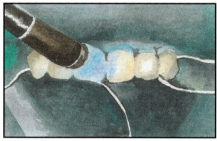 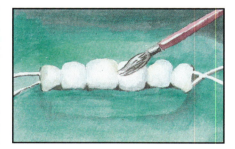

After this power bleaching process, some initial sensitivity may be felt, but commonly subsides by the evening, returning to normal by the next day. The amount of sensitivity varies from person to person and everyone has different pain thresholds.

People who have already very sensitive teeth may prefer to spread out the whole process over several visits for the same effect. However immediately after each bleaching session, you must not expose your teeth to substances which quickly stain them namely, tobacco, tea, coffee, red wine, and so on. These should also be avoided or reduced if you wish the whiteness to last longer. The result of in-office bleaching is often dramatic. Teeth can look very whitened immediately afterwards and they can remain so for 1-3 years, to a lifetime. It's so popular because it works and is never regretted afterwards. It is important to realize that the bleaching of teeth with these chemicals can only bring out the full potential whiteness of the natural teeth, and cannot be expected to compare with the absolute whiteness offered by a porcelain veneer or crown. The advantage of vital tooth bleaching is that many teeth in the mouth can be whitened together at a fraction of the cost.

Darkly Stained Teeth

Discoloured dark teeth are commonly caused by the tetracycline group of antibiotic medicines taken during childhood in the previous generation. However doctors now no longer prescribe tetracycline medicines for the children of today, and such tooth dark teeth caused by it would be no longer common in the new generation.

Less commonly it is due to fluorosis, a condition caused by the overexposure to or over-ingestion of fluoride mineral during the growing years. In some parts of the world where the water supply contains fluoride in a concentration of up to 6 parts per million, (or 6ppm, or >6 times the safer level of <1ppm in areas with water fluoridation) fluorosis will occur for those born or grew up in the area. Their teeth become severely darkened in colour. The swallowing of fluoride tablets and fluoride drops, given to young children in an attempt to protect their teeth from tooth decay may also end up grossly darken their growing teeth. The direct topical application of fluoride on already erupted teeth is far safer then by ingestion. (Very rarely tooth discolouration may be due to the abnormal formation of the enamel or dentine). There is little else to do for darkly stained teeth, and as tooth bleaching cannot improve them satisfactorily, the only real solution for them is by veneering or crowning them all with porcelain material.

Teeth with dead nerves inside, caused by decay or fractured by trauma, if left untreated would produce decomposing blood pigments which stain the tooth. After treatment, the tooth could be bleached inside before placing a porcelain jacket crown.

Porcelain Veneers

Veneers are wafer-thin laminates that are bonded directly to the fronts of teeth, rather like the artificial fingernail laminates. These are glued to the front surfaces of the front teeth. These are useful for closing gaps between teeth, for restoring completely worn enamel surfaces caused by excessive toothbrushing, fractured corners of front teeth, or commonly for disguising the discoloured front teeth which never responded well to tooth bleaching. It is very popular nowadays.

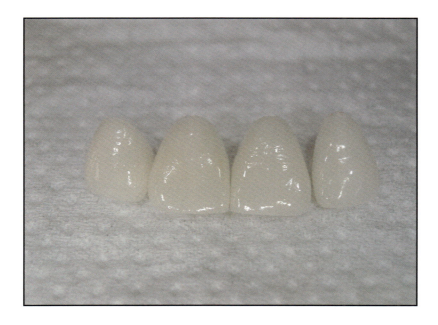

Porcelain veneers do not stain easily, and the surface shine is retained almost indefinitely. They are beautiful and natural looking when crafted by the hands of a skilled technician. Porcelain is capable of replicating natural teeth effectively but they should never be made one at a time as it can be very difficult to match exactly the shade of an individual veneer to the other existing ones. It is always best to make several veneers simultaneously to obtain the most uniform smile in terms of exact colour and positional accuracy. Later additions to your smile may not match exactly and any alterations of the shade and porcelain layerings can make the individual newly installed veneer look odd. Veneers can be applied for mildly malpositioned teeth improving their alignment. This may be a short-cut method to improve the appearance of slightly crooked teeth in lieue of orthodontics, e. g. minor tooth rotations, imbalanced crown lengths. The placement of veneers must be precisional since incomplete seating, or press-fit of the veneers onto the front surfaces of teeth could increase the overall thickness of the front teeth, bulging the lips out. Veneers are positioned such that you cannot bite onto them directly as they can be chipped off. Porcelain is brittle and veneers are thin, repairs for chipped porcelain is either difficult or impossible and they would need to be wholly replaced. The lower front teeth must always bite behind the upper teeth, avoiding any heavy direct contacts at the incisor edges. If you have a protruded bite, your lower jaw being out further than your upper jaw, you may not be a suitable candidate for veneers because your lower teeth may just shear them off. The same applies if you tend to brux or grind at your teeth. You must have enough back teeth to bite on otherwise all the chewing forces are aimed at the front wafer-thin veneers. Never use your beautiful veneers to nibble on nuts or sunflower seeds. They will chip easily if you use them in this way. Biting an apple is perhaps OK, but I would avoid it if I were you. I simply couldn't guarantee it.

Porcelain Jacket Crowns

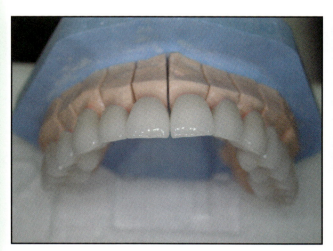
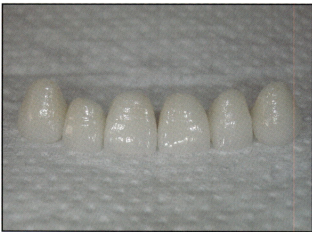

Whereas veneers are thin half to one millimeter laminates glued permanently to the fronts of teeth to mask their discolouration, they could be sheared off by your bite. Sometimes their thin structure is too translucent and cannot sufficiently mask the dark discolourations. if the tooth is too heavily stained. Porcelain crowns can be made with thicker porcelain to provide a more effective masking. However, more of the tooth is filed down in order to accommodate them, at least 1 mm all the way around.

The difference between porcelain veneers and porcelain crowns is that veneers are like half-crowns, or facings, whereas crowns are the full jacket versions which would require more tooth structure to be filed, i. e. circumferentially.

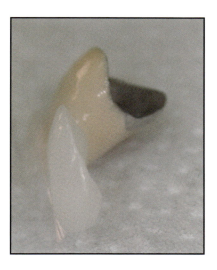

Veneer Vs. Crown.

Treatment Sequence.

Several sessions are needed for making porcelain veneers and crowns. The filings and fittings are all done under a local anaesthetic. After filing, a mold is taken of your teeth which would be sent to the dental laboratory for fabrication.

Immediately temporary crowns or veneers are provided for you for the waiting period as it may take 2 weeks before they are finished from the laboratory. The temporary teeth are usually made of white plastic, and can be easily stained. Avoid staining foods, especially the gravy from curries which could immediately stain the temporary teeth bright yellow.

Beverages and tobacco are fine, but do not drink anything too hot or cold as the teeth are slightly sensitive during this temporary period. Brush at the gums and teeth as best you can, remembering to keep those gum lines especially clean.

Temporary crowns are often poorly adapted to the teeth and may collect more dental plaque.

The colour of the porcelain can be matched either by your dentist, or together with yourself, if you wish to play an active role in the shade taking process. There are often various shades in every natural tooth, and a complete blank white colour for any porcelain crown or veneer can look too unnatural. Porcelain teeth should not be too glossy, they should have some texture.

Opting for a one white colour could look fine, but as like the white tiles on the kitchen wall, it could make your smile looking fake and artificial. Teeth are generally slightly yellower near to the gum line, and progressively whiten towards the edge. Sometimes the very edges of front teeth can have some translucencies of half to one millimeter. As far as the shape and form is concerned, crowns and veneers must never be bulky. For the front teeth, they should be tucked in just under your gum line, without any edges showing as you flash your gums. The worst thing that can happen is to have all the porcelains looking great, but at the gums you can see their black margins where the crowns fit. In cosmetic dentistry, it is not just about crowns being done to improve your smile, but it has more to do with how masterfully they can be done to achieve the most pleasing and natural smile everyone wished they were born with. One of the greatest assets that a person can ever have is a smile that displays beautiful, natural-looking teeth, even if they were all artificial. Metal bonded porcelain crowns can tend to show up at the gum line exposing those metallic black margins as the gum recede with age. However porcelain jacket crowns are less obvious and are better blended to the tooth even after gums recede, since they are devoid of all metallic structures underneath.

The worst-looking porcelain crown you can have is one that shows a huge black line at the gums, the crown is too bulbous, the colour is too solid and lifeless, and the colour does not even match the tooth beside it.

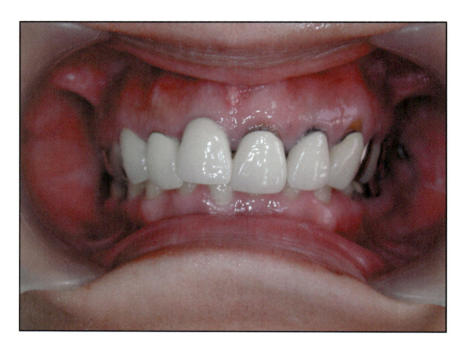

Exposed Black Margins.

Colour.

Colour is probably the most complex artistic element and dependent on a vast amount of other external factors. Teeth consist of a multitude of colours, being generally browner at the gum line where the enamel is thinner. For an artificial tooth to look natural, it takes a combination of many shades to form the natural aesthetics. Flat white crowns look like a mouthful of kitchen tiles.

Colours are far more critical when it is to exactly match the natural tooth next to it. Canines are generally slightly yellower than the incisors. Young people will have lighter teeth with more translucencies, and older people will tend to have more yellow to brown solid coloured teeth, showing less translucency and with less surface texture. The enamel is worn smooth over the years with toothbrushing, and the teeth edges are worn flat after many decades of chewing.

People with darker complexions tend to make their teeth look lighter because of the increased contrast. Similarly women can enhance the apparent lightness of their teeth by the use of darker shades of make-up or lipsticks. Increasing the contrast between the teeth and the facial surroundings can create the illusion of having whiter teeth. Whiter teeth is generally more attractive and it is often associated with youth and vitality.

Gaps Between Front Teeth.

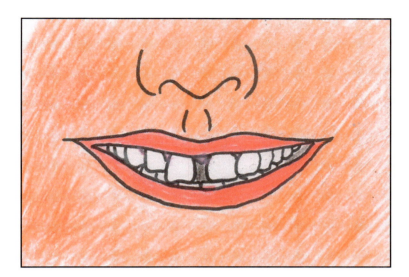

"Huge gaps between the two front teeth can be particularly distracting to any observer".

A gap between the two front teeth is known as a midline diastema. If there is only a small gap between your two front teeth, they could both simply be veneered or crowned with porcelain material to close the gap permanently. If, however, the gap is too big and wide, it would need to be closed with orthodontic treatment, and all the teeth on either side of the midline are moved in to close the midline space. A gap between the two front teeth is sometimes caused by the very thick gumflesh between them, or on rare occasions, there is a small extra tooth high up in the gums wedged between them at their roots. Whether gumflesh or extra-tooth (supernumary), both are ideally surgically removed before the gap is closed. If the gap is very small, it could be filled in with two individual side white fillings using composite resin material.

Reshaping Teeth.

If the front surfaces of the teeth is very rough, it could be easily polished by your dentist using special polishing techniques known as microabrasion, and macroabrasion. Corners of the teeth which have been chipped could also be rounded off to feel smoother. If the edges of your two front teeth are not balanced, one tooth appearing longer than the other, a fine abrasive disc can be used to level the longer one slightly to make them both equal. If however, the front tooth is particularly too small, as like a peg-shape tooth, it could be improved with a porcelain jacket crown, or a porcelain veneer.

Correcting Occlusion.

The term "occlusion" describes the way in which teeth bite, or occlude together, and a bad bite is termed a mal-occlusion.

If the teeth are not biting correctly caused by fillings, crowns or bridges, these can be reshaped to allow the teeth on both sides of the mouth to touch simultaneously as the teeth bite together. If you leave your teeth to bite in disharmony, the jaws may compensate for this by deviating to one side as the mouth closes. This causes unnatural strain on the jaw muscles, and leads to facial muscle pains. The jawjoints also begin to click each time the mouth opens or closes. Teeth which had been extracted and left unreplaced over time will allow other teeth to tilt and shift into the void, disturbing the balance of the bite.

An orthodontist can correct this by repositioning those teeth which had shifted, back into their previous positions. After this is achieved, the missing tooth or teeth can be replaced.

Alternatively a good dentist, or a prosthodontist can help you to reshape or rebuild your teeth to improve your bite quickly.

18. Cosmetic Restorations

Bad dentalworks can ruin your smile! Their quality, colour, form and integrity are all determining.

Once damages had been allowed to occur to teeth, their repair or replacement treatments require artificial materials to be used. Not only are these materials ever quite as good as the original, natural tooth structures, but the health of the repaired tooth and the gums around them are never quite the same afterwards. There is no available method to date which is able to regenerate tooth structures. Although "test-tube teeth" aims promisingly towards this objective through stem cell research, it is still at its very early stages. The materials used to restore teeth can affect your smile cosmetically. However, if they deteriorate in the mouth over time, they can deteriorate your smile at the same time. Some materials are more durable than others and gold shines in this respect, but gold and silver coloured fillings have declined in recent years because of their colour.

White fillings are either made of composite resin or porcelain. Now when compared, composite resin fillings are never as strong as porcelains and are best limited to small cavities. Composite resin fillings are however much cheaper and can be done directly in a single visit at the chairside. Porcelain, on the other hand, is far more expensive and is made indirectly at the dental laboratory from a mold taken of your teeth. Whereas a composite resin filling tends to stain both on and around it over time, particularly around their edges, porcelain is however, harder, far more durable and more resistant to staining in the long term. A porcelain inlay is like a piece of a jigsaw puzzle, made of china ware, tailored to fit accurately into that one specific cavity in your tooth and will not fit any other tooth cavity in your mouth nor any other's in the whole world. Composite resin on the other hand is fluid, blended into any cavity like a soft white piece of plastercine, shaped to an approximation by hand instruments, and hardened by a chemical reaction. This is triggered by exposure to a light source. During this hardening process, it also tends to shrink slightly, leaving that tiny micro-crevice around its perimeter which may eventually collect stains. However the effect is less significant in the small cavity, but if you should need a white filling for the large cavity, a porcelain inlay is more appropriate.

The art of cosmetic dentistry involves not only restoring your teeth to full health, but also aims to retain the appearance of your smile in its most natural form. A smile which displays the black margins of your crown and filling edges, gaps under your porcelain bridge, or metal clasps of your denture could never be aesthetic. Crown margins are best tucked just under the gum line, porcelain bridges are adapted exactly to the gum ridges, and denture clasps are redesigned and positioned discreetly.

Whilst cosmetic dentistry is concerned with correct colours which can serve to camouflage their existence, the fine quality of restorations in the mouth determines the long term survival of the teeth they aim to preserve. They should all feel smooth and comfortable when they are in the mouth and the precision of their fit is of the highest degree. Their shapes, forms, contours, and sizes should replicate the lost tissues in order to restore teeth back to their original anatomy, to maintain their original contacts with all neighboring and opposing teeth. The more perfect they are, the more comfortable, durable and "invisible" they get.

The reason why dental restorations which are indirectly fabricated from a model of your cavities in the dental laboratory often last longer is because the technician is able to contour them precisely. Fillings which are directly made at the chair side and placed into cavities by hand may not give the dentist the luxury of time and the 360 degree view provided by a model, and the approximate shaping of them at the chair side often can result in oversized fillings which overflow outside of the cavities to form either overhanging ledges, or undersized fillings which fail to fill the cavity completely, creating step-defects around their perimeters. Such ill-fitting and poorly constructed restorations not only looks bad, but they invite food and dental plaque to settle around them to cause recurrent decay, drastically shortening the longevity of the tooth. Blackness around fillings could ruin your smile. The "perfect filling" with perfect fittings do still have fine margins at their edges where they meet the tooth and can still invite the collection of dental plaque, but far less. Once you need to have artificial materials in the mouth, it becomes inescapably important that they and all of their many perimeters are swept clean at all times because their existence alone creates new stagnation areas for extra dental plaque to collect. This is why the gums around crowns tend to bleed more readily than around natural teeth, and fillings tend to have more recurrences of decay underneath them when compared with wholly intact and natural teeth without fillings (virgin teeth), in the same mouth.

A Mouthful Of Problems.

If you do have too many large patchy fillings at your front teeth, all done in composite resins, are tatty and stained, and your teeth are all intrinsically discoloured, you could choose to have them all either veneered, or even all crowned using porcelain.

Veneering or crowning your complete smile is never justified unless you are honestly disturbed by the way your teeth look, and their discolouration is so appalling that all the other treatments, like tooth-bleaching, had all been tried and failed.

Veneers and crowns, all done in porcelain, is rather expensive but it could be the ultimate solution for you. It is important to discuss this with your dentist just in case there are other alternatives to solve your particular problems. The other advantage of veneering or crowning front teeth is that their mildly crooked arrangements could be improved, and these could straighten your smile for you. If the front teeth are slightly rotated, if their shapes and forms are small or irregular, or if their surfaces are heavily banded, rough and pitted with horizontal rings of stainings, these would all be corrected in the process. Sometimes even a slightly lop-sided smile could be straightened by crowning teeth alone, and also mid-line shifts could be better improved.

The neatest restoration that can exist in your mouth is when it does not appear to exist at all, to any observer. Porcelain can achieve this, but it must be crafted with skill and care. Natural shades of colours are blended to mimic the natural looks of tooth substances, and the shapes and forms of the restorations are sculptured to duplicate the natural anatomy of teeth.

Their edges are never in plain view, and their finest precision fittings allow the tooth to appear completely natural and intact.

It is important to recognize that, though obvious as it is, whenever we require to have artificial materials in the mouth, their imperfections alone could have adverse influences on the health and beauty of our smile. Dentures must be stable and click well into their correct positions. They may, however, show their metal hooks if there are only the front teeth left for them to hook onto. This may not be the best situation for them and this can sometimes be improved by positioning the hooks nearer to the gum line, rather than positioned half-way up. If dentures cannot offer you acceptable aesthetics, especially if they show the metal hooks, you may option to have your missing teeth replaced with the use of Dental Implants.

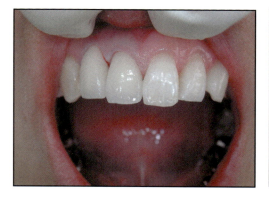
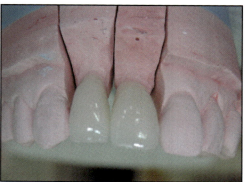

19. GUMMY SMILES

In approximately 30% of people, they have short upper lips, resulting in a high lip-line.

LIP-LINES:

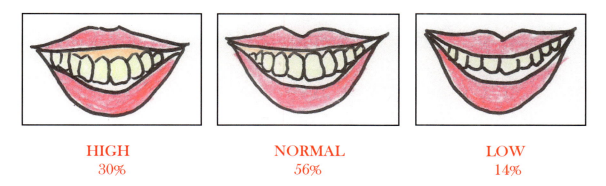

| HIGH | NORMAL | LOW |
| 30% | 56% | 14% |

Sometimes the teeth are just too short, and there is simply more of the gums than teeth. People who have high lip-lines would simply display this disproportional situation more readily, in which case it bothers them.

This appearance can be easily improved by doing a gingivectomy, or a gum-lift. The whole procedure can be done within an hour. By removing some of the excess gums above the gum line, at the necks of teeth, the gum line can be effectively moved up by 2.0 mm. As a result more of the teeth can be exposed to proportion correctly with the gums. As the roots of the teeth are now showing, porcelain crowns or porcelain veneers can be fitted onto the teeth to include the root areas. This recontours their proportions for a better smile. This technique is also known as crown lengthening.

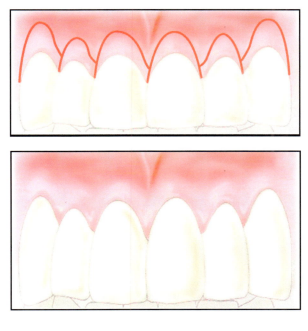

CROWN LENGTHENING.

20. Bad Breath-You Are Always The Last Person To Know

Bad breath, also known scientifically as halitosis, or oral malodour, describes obvious unpleasant odours from your breath.

What causes bad breath? Most people who have it never even realized it themselves until quite embarrassingly, a colleague, a close friend, or a spouse, finally tells them of the bad news! Women actually get very upset about if her husband had always known it all along but had never spoken a word. Well we cannot smell our own breaths and besides, we are probably so accustomed to our own smell that we would never realize it. Serious bad breath can actually be very offensive and it can affect us socially. A fresh clean breath, on the other hand, can be attractive and appealing during conversations and intimate moments.

What Causes Bad Breath?

Temporary bad breath is the common temporary type caused by eating certain foods such as garlic, onions, certain fruits like papaya or durian, or the dry mouth with lots of plaque in the morning can produce bad breath. However these causes are tackled simply by brushing the teeth, using mouthwash, or by chewing minty gums.

Persistent bad breath on the other hand is more lingering and it affects nearly a quarter of the people at large. Bad breath can have adverse effects on one's personal and business relationships, leading to a lowered sense of well-being and personal pride.

Personal stress emerges within oneself. Heavy smoking and a poor level of oral hygiene is often to blame. More seriously it could be a mouthful of gum disease with rotting flesh, or tooth decay with grossly rotten teeth and broken roots all heavily infested with bacteria and pus. The discharge of pus within the mouth can produce such a foul odour which can be so repulsive that it can make an impact on others. A face-to-face talk with full exposure to the foul breath is so highly off-putting, the gossip can degenerate one's self-image and pride. Some medical conditions can also cause bad breath such as diabetes, or uraemia, which have distinctive odours. Long term courses of antibiotics can disturb bacterial balance in the stomach and gut, killing off too many good essential bacterias and disturbing the normal bacterial balance. The long term use of broad spectrum antibiotics such as the Tetracyclines or the Penicillins, can allow fungal infections to flourish freely which can cause odours. Yogurt foods may be included in the daily diet to help replenish the good bacteria perished by the antibiotics. Salivary gland diseases reduces saliva production, and a constant dry mouth will encourage more bacteria to grow in the mouth. People who need to take a lot of medicines will tend to have less saliva in the mouth, as a common side effect, as also those who had recently received head and neck radiation treatments. However, in general bad breath does increase with age. All sorts of mouth infections can arise from the lack of saliva, and tooth decay start to creep up typically at the necks of teeth, also known as root-decay. A good way to illustrate this is to imagine if your eyes failed to produce tears, if for whatever reason the tear glands were damaged. Dry-eyes will result in infections which will result in conjunctivitis. Stomach diseases producing frequent regurgitation of stomach acids, (as in vomiting) will give bad breath.

Worms?!

Parasites living in the gut, (or helminthic infections), could also be a cause of bad breath but it is not uncommon nowadays because we all like to eat undercooked meat and other raw foods. We could have worms living in us and we would never suspect it; they could come from the raw fish, raw beef, we've eaten. Testing for parasites is good but these tests are often unreliable. If you tend to consume raw foods frequently, you might consider to take a simple general anti-parasite medicine once a year, such as a single tablet of 500mg Mebendazole which can readily be prescribed to you by your doctor without the absolute need for a test. It rules out most of the worms you are likely to encounter.

The Tongue

Presently true bad breath is not well-understood except that for the most part they are considered caused by the foods we eat, or the bacteria in our mouths. The tongue can trap a great deal of bacteria and scraping the tongue with quality tongue scrapers may be helpful. The mouth is certainly a safe-haven for bacteria, as like our whole gastro-intestinal system, but the oral flora is often well balanced enough not to cause problems. There are hundreds of types of bacteria in our mouths, some are harmless, but several scores of these can become potentially harmful if left unchecked by our immune system, and these reside at the back of the tongue and near the soft palate. The tongue surface is rough at the back and will allow the bacteria to mingle with the collection of dead cells, dead bacteria, bits of food particles, and they will ferment all sorts of odoured chemicals such as hydrogen sulphide which would make your breath smell like a rotten egg.

Testing For Bad Breath

You can never notice your own bad breath by breathing out and smelling it through your nose. Try these:

1. Lick the back of your hand and smell it afterwards.
2. Use a spoon to scrape the back of the tongue and smell that.
3. Floss between some of your teeth, then smell the floss.
4. Ask a family member to smell your breath.

Management.

Mouthwashes, freshening mints, mouth sprays, toothbrushing can all give you remarkable improvements. Bad breath may be further reduced by using special formulated hydrogen peroxide mouthrinses. Brushing and flossing after meals is useful to remove rotting food fragments from between the teeth, and cleaning the tongue surface with a tongue scraper is very helpful. Have a thorough dental check up and ask your dentist to look for any infections in the mouth, or any other explainable causes. Chewing sugarless gum, like xylitol, can help to increase saliva in the mouth which kills bacteria, to combat bad breath. Always drink plenty of water and if all else fails, go for a microbiological testing at the hospital. Swabbing a sample of teeth, the tongue and all oral tissues may help to identify any unusual types of bacteria. An ENT (Ear, nose, throat) specialist may be another person who can help you, but in any case include a general medical check-up to identify or eliminate any general medical conditions which may be the cause of your bad breath.

21. Food For Teeth

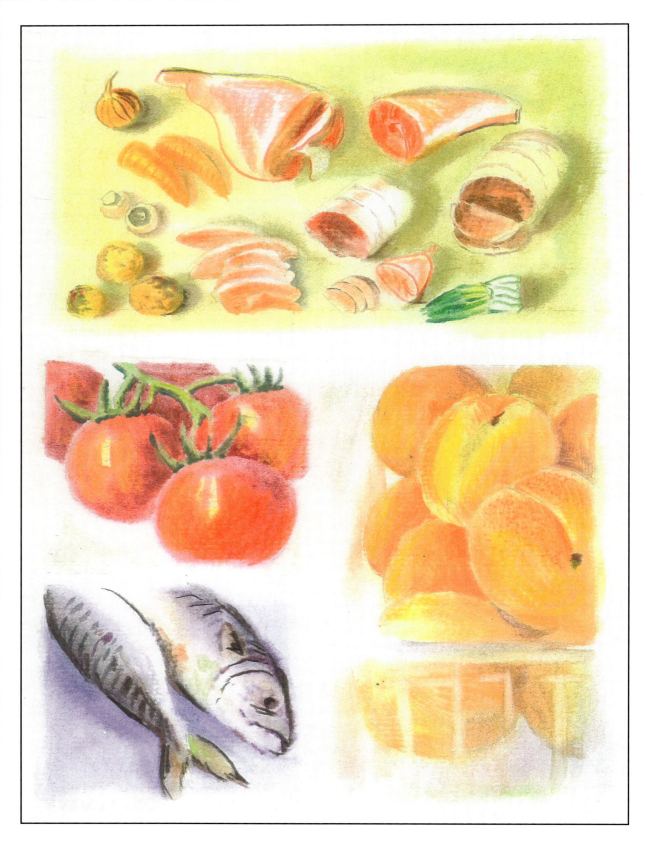

Nutrition And Dental Health.

A healthy overall smile is determined by our general health and nutritional status. The soft tissue cells of our mouths are continually shedding and reforming like our skin, and require a constant supply of nutrients. When this constant supply is reduced, symptoms quickly develop and manifest itself in the mouth. Anaemia is a good example when the low levels of iron results in smooth, red tongues (glossitis). Mouth ulcers also occur with iron deficiency and women are commoner to suffer this. There may also be signs of fungal infections in the mouth and at the corners of the lips which become red and sore (angular cheilitis). If the mouth feels dry, always drink plenty of water to keep the oral tissues moist. People who take a lot of medicines tend to have less saliva and this makes them more prone to mouth infections. The health of the bones and teeth are more dependent on calcium and other minerals. A glass of milk a day could supply you with one-third of your daily calcium needs.

Vitamins And Minerals.

Vitamin A:

Vitamin A is important in the process of tooth formation.

Vitamin A comes from animal sources, such as eggs, meat, milk, cheese, cream, liver, kidney, cod, and halibut fish oil.

Vitamin B2:

Deficiency of this vitamin B2, or riboflavin, may result in soreness of the mouth, lips, tongue, and cracks at the corners of the lips. The mouth feels like burning, but is reversed when the vitamin is consumed. This vitamin is also important for healthy hair, nails and skin but too much alcohol and coffee can destroy it.

Good sources of this vitamin includes milk, liver, eggs, meat, green vegetables and fish.

Vitamin B12 & Folic Acid:

These are vital for the repair and replacement of cells, and deficiency results in soreness of all soft tissues.

Mouth ulcers may develop as any break in the skin surfaces of the mouth will find difficulty to repair itself without these vitamins.

Good sources for these include liver, beef, milk, cheese, eggs, green vegetables, fresh oranges, wheat germ.

Vitamin C:

Vitamin C is most important for the formation of the underlying connective tissues that hold the gums together.

Deficiency of vitamin C results in "scurvy", and in the presence of dental plaque, the gums begin to bleed and deteriorate rapidly, causing teeth to eventually loosen. Vitamin C is very protective in gum disease because it has a lot to do with the synthesis of collagen. The fibres which attach teeth to the bone is made of collagen. In addition, vitamin C has also antibacterial effects. Vitamin C is required everyday and fresh citrus fruits are the best sources. It is water soluble and easily excreted from the body and so it must be consumed everyday.

Vitamin D:

Vitamin D regulates Calcium and Phosphorus, maintaining normal teeth and jawbones. It also reduces the loss of bone around teeth. Good sources include fish-liver oils, milk, butter, dairy products, and exposure of the skin to sunshine will allow the human body to produce vitamin D by itself. Staying indoors 24 hours a day will deny you of this important feature. Even an hour of facial, arm or leg exposure to natural sunlight is beneficial and vitamin D can help your body to absorb more calcium.

Vitamin E:

Vitamin E is an antioxidant that protects body tissue from damage caused by unstable substances called free radicals. Free radicals can harm cells, tissues, and organs, and they are believed to be one of the causes of the degenerative processes seen in aging. Vitamin E is also important in the formation of red blood cells . Vitamin E is found in the following foods; Wheat germ, Corn Nuts, Seeds, Olives, Spinach and other green leafy vegetables, Asparagus.

Vitamin E may help to reduce the toxic effects of the mercury in the amalgam fillings which contain approximately 50% of mercury (Hg). Vitamin E can help to protect the body from any heavy metal toxicity.

Calcium:

Optimal calcium is essential to the developing teeth and bones. Just ensure that you are indeed not deficient.

Sufficient intake of calcium also protects against osteoporosis, strengthening the jaws and prevents tooth-loss.

In some studies, it was shown that women who had osteoporosis before the age of 40 resulted in early tooth loss, compared with normal women after the age of 40. The more teeth they lost, the less bone they had also in their spine, wrist, and hips, which became susceptible to fractures. However calcium is also regulated by the presence of Vitamin D, and the parathyroid hormones, so the over-surplus intake of calcium is not necessarily more beneficial. Milk, cheese and dairy products are good sources.

Magnesium:

The balance of magnesium and calcium is important for normal growths. A deficiency of magnesium may lead to swollen and sore gums, but these heal up when sufficient intake is included in our diets.

Phosphorus:

This is an essential part of our enamel and dentine, and is important during the formation of the teeth.

Adequate amounts should be taken by the mother during pregnancy, and later taken by the infant throughout the growing years, and beyond. The balance between calcium and phosphorus is essential for the normal formation of bones and teeth.

Chewing raw fruits and vegetables can help to scrape the teeth and reduce the accumulation of dental plaque.

Balanced Diets.

Generally a good balanced diet, with adequate proteins, fruits and vegetables, bananas, whole grain, bread, chicken, fish, meats, cereals, vitamin D-fortified and low-fat milk, natural sunlight, cheese and yogurt, will be quite adequate.

Avoid tobacco, sticky sweets, and sucking on citrus fruits, do not take sugary snacks just before bedtime. A high standard maintenance of oral hygiene will enhance the life expectancy of your teeth.

22. Things You Should Know About BRUSHING

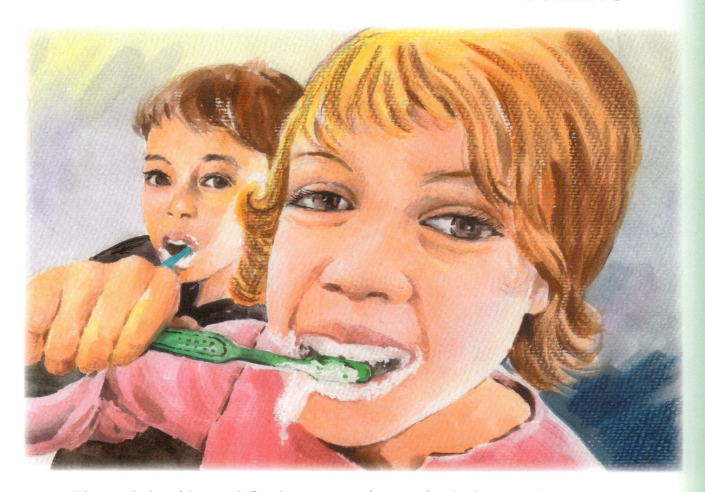

Thorough brushing and flossing your teeth everyday is the most important routine to perfect as new bacteria forms on your teeth each day. Apart from cleaning the teeth themselves, the bacteria must also be removed from the gum lines. Spending 3 minutes on brushing and 3 minutes on flossing, twice a day could save you a lot of problems. A sound oral hygiene regimen protects you from cavities and gum disease. In a recent study published in the American Journal of Dentistry it was calculated that a person's brushing time was just 37 seconds, and further studies revealed that only 20% of people regularly performed acceptable flossing, while there was also over-whelming evidence to suggest that a substantial part of the population never floss at all. This is alarming news for all dentists.

The Gum Line.

The gums serve to wrap themselves around the necks of the teeth just above the bone to form a tight seal. There is a tiny space between the gums and the teeth known as the gingival sulcus (or sulcus), and normally it is about 2mm deep. This forms a normal pocket but is a common source of infection. Once the pocket deepens beyond 4mm, as caused by the toxins of the bacteria, it is known as a pathological pocket. This gum seal at the base of the sulcus must remain intact as it forms your defence barrier which separates the sterile (root) and non-sterile (crown) parts of the tooth. This is your first line of defence and the initial gum-seal is rather like the cork-seal in a wine bottle, or the protective seal of the zipped plastic bag. Dental plaque remaining along this gum line produces toxins which will destroy and breach this gum seal, creating an opening to penetrate inwards. Once they sink their way in beneath this cuff they will disintegrate every fibre connection of the tooth roots to the bone. When the tooth root is entirely covered in tartar and bacteria, no living cells would survive and remain attached to it, leaving a space containing dead cells around it. This leakage not only allows bacteria inside to become virtually impossible for you to remove with your toothbrush but it also becomes an open gateway for an unlimited supply of fresh bacteria to enter in and "join the party".

This destructive process is painless and will go on happily "behind your back". If it was allowed to remain unchecked by professionals, the tooth will eventually loosen and shed. There is actually a battle going on here because you do have some defence cells (or your soldiers) to fight them off for you, but it depends on the state of your health and nutrition. The teeth are attached by collagen fibres to our jawbones, and vitamin C does play an important role in maintaining collagen health. On the other hand, a total lack of this vitamin, as in scurvy, can result in more gum bleedings and tooth losses. Smoking has adverse effects on the gums, and the gum healing amidst tobacco is far less efficient.

The rate, extent and amount of your gums being destroyed by your enemy bacteria is resisted by your ability to send good strong soldiers into the battle for your defence. Our bodies are always in constant battle with all sorts of harmful invaders which is why some people have more problems than others, and it is the fittest who will always survive.

CLEANING STAGNATION AREAS.

Dental plaque also tends to hide in the stagnation areas of your teeth, such as the in-between areas of the back teeth, crooked teeth, wisdom teeth, around the prominent edges of fillings, crowns, dentures, orthodontic brackets, and the naturally formed deep pits and fissures of teeth. If these are missed by your cleanings, they will simply accumulate, form lactic acids with sugar and cause cavities.

DANGER ZONES.

Dentists see things differently from patients, dentists are interested in the danger zones, namely the back teeth, the areas between them, the areas behind them, and the wisdom teeth areas. Dentists also focus on the condition of the gums. Patients rarely observe their gums. They focus mostly on the fronts of front teeth, occasionally the back teeth, but never between or behind them. The points of view are often quite the opposite. Cleaning teeth is like polishing shoes, it must be completely thorough to include the front, back and side surfaces. Similarly, cleaning teeth includes flossing their sides.

As the old saying goes, "You only floss the teeth you wish to keep".

RELEARNING.

As we already know that brushing and flossing is important but it may be useful to wonder for a moment why we should take plaque so seriously. For starters, once we've realized that dental plaque caused people to have fillings and gum diseases which alone virtually created the whole of the Dental Industry we might be more weary of it, or at least give it some respect. In order to illustrate for understanding better the rationale behind brushing, it would be a good idea for you to first take a quick glimpse at your own teeth in the mirror. If you have any fillings in your teeth, they are mainly caused by plaque. . not sugar. . but plaque, the scientifically proven no. 1 culprit. Sugar alone is not capable to produce the lactic acids which cause cavities. To demonstrate this, if you happen to have an extracted tooth, (e. g. a baby tooth which shed out), brush it clean, dry it and smear a lot of chocolate on it. Display it in a glass bottle on your shelf. You won't find it ever forming any cavities on that tooth no matter how long you wait as the "plaque factor" is missing.

Would you remember all the injections and drillings you had to go through when you got those fillings? Well these fillings are all likely to need replacements in the future, even if you brush well from now on, because fillings can deteriorate over time.

Dental plaque is basically a sticky white film of bacteria that forms on tooth surfaces every single day, and continuously throughout the day, and sits on your gum lines to cause all your problems. It is an unnoticeable yet ongoing process which never ceases, second-by- second even as we speak. The only good news is that removing it all once a day suffices to limit its harm, the aim is to Reset to "0000" the oral plaque level at the beginning of each day. If everyone was 100% meticulous with their brushing, flossing, and so on, successfully eliminating every speck of plaque from their gums and teeth, they could save for themselves a lot of money and suffering. Dentists spend their careers repairing the tooth damages caused by daily plaque.

If the rate of formation of plaque is not well-balanced by its efficient removal, the resulting accumulation will gain the upper hand to cause problems.

We've all learnt to brush our teeth every morning and night since we were little, but how many of us really know that we are doing it all correctly? It seems such a basic task but yet few people actually do it right. Your dentist or hygienist are the best people to give you advice on this daily routine, and sessions spent with them for relearning this is always worthwhile.

Most people don't know how to floss their teeth, and if they did have many bridgeworks in their mouths, flossing under them is often "rarely done". Afterall, it is troublesome. Flossing does become more critical for those with a mouthful of many large fillings, crowns and bridges .

Once artificial materials are permanently attached in the mouth, it becomes inescapably important that they and all of their many edges and seams are swept clean at all times because their existence alone creates new stagnation areas for plaque. The existence of their many seams is the very reason why the gums around them tend to bleed more readily and fillings tend to have more recurrences of decay underneath, resulting in their need for replacements from time to time. Healthy teeth completely intact without fillings, also known as virgin teeth, are seamless.

The Morning Rush.

The main reason why brushing in the morning is so important is because plaque forms most abundantly during sleeping.

During the rest of the day, the salivary flow disturbs their formations. There is less saliva during sleep, which explains why our mouths are so dry whenever we wake up. It's better to brush and floss before breakfast rather than after because the bacteria are then eliminated from the teeth before sugar enters the mouth. Have a good rinse of the mouth before you leave for work, and do not chew on a candy bar on the way to the bus stop. The trouble with morning brushing is that people are very hurried to go to school or to work and have less time to do it properly. A second

attempt before bedtime makes up for the morning rush.
"BRUSH YOUR TEETH BEFORE BREAKFAST, RATHER THAN AFTER. . ."

The Significance Of Good Oral Hygiene.

We need to clean our teeth because the number of bacteria in the mouth is immense and their variety beyond exacting figures.

Damage to our precious teeth and gums is mostly due to the presence of bacteria on the teeth and gums. Sugar alone causes no harm as organic acids cannot form without plaque and gums are never damaged without their toxins.

A common misconception is that pregnancy, vitamin C deficiency (as in scurvy), or if one has a family history of gum disease, the gums must deteriorate. One has "weaker gums" so to speak. Gum abscesses start to appear, there's more bleeding, and everything seems to go downhill. However, scientifically speaking, these other factors are unable to manifest their untoward influences on gum tissues in a plaque-free mouth. In all such described statuses, the gums merely over-react to the presence of plaque due to a lowered body resistance. The inflammation they trigger is amplified and is therefore destructive.

Stepping-up the oral hygiene will counteract all such adverse effects when the body is less capable to defend itself.

Similarly people in poor health, such as suffering from diabetes, and are malnourished do have very rapidly destructive gum disease because the gums deteriorate even with the slightest traces of plaque in the mouth. We are constantly living in balance with bacteria and although we are unable to remove every bacteria from our mouths, with extra efforts we could nevertheless attempt to remove a greater proportion of them. This way we can rely less on our body defense capabilities.

So what exactly is plaque ?

Within seconds of tooth brushing a thin layer of salivary protein (mainly glycoprotein) is deposited evenly onto the tooth surface, including on the fillings, dentures, orthodontic brackets and so on. This layer is called the pellicle. It is smooth, and colourless, and is approximately half a micron in thickness. It is initially free of bacteria and adsorbs onto tooth surfaces possibly due to an electrostatic affinity between the tooth surface and the glycoprotein. This thin film of pellicle is in itself very harmless, but in fact beneficial because it contains a supply of salivary calcium and phosphate which are essential minerals for teeth. Its binding to the tooth surface is quite firm and cannot be washed away by irrigation with mouthwash or water. It must be removed by positive friction, as by toothbrushing, flossing, or chewing and all such similar mechanical methods. Within minutes after the pellicle has been formed on teeth, it is populated by bacteria. In thin layers it is not immediately visible. It forms preferentially in sheltered areas of the mouth, such as between the teeth, around the fillings, crowns, under the bridges, dentures, around orthodontic brackets, on "already present" tartar and at the gum line. The plaque grows by internal multiplication plus surface deposition.

In thick layers, it turns yellower in colour, seen as a gelatinous soft thick film which can be readily removed by a toothbrush or even scraped off with your fingernail. Dental plaque is soft and so it is never necessary to scrub your teeth heavily with a hard toothbrush. You can easily see it every morning before you brush, just use you fingernail and scrape on your front tooth.

Dental plaque which is not removed by your brushing and flossing will remain there to form tartar within a week or two, and once it's formed you can't even scrape it off with a fork ! This is why a regular scale and polish is so imperative.

So What Exactly Is Tartar ?

Dental calculus, or tartar is the stony crust that forms on teeth, and appears similar to the crust commonly found inside of kettles in countries which provide hard drinking water. Tartar is calcified dental plaque, or plaque enriched with calcium phosphate.

It is rarely found on baby or adult teeth of children under the age of 9, but after this age, it starts to form abundantly.

In reality nearly all adults have some tartar in their mouths and these cannot be removed by themselves. They must be removed regularly by dental professionals with suitable instruments. It appears light yellow at first, but is later heavily stained by tea, coffee, tobacco, betel nut, or red wine. Whereas tartar on teeth above the gum line is easily removed by special instruments, those found deeper on the roots of teeth below the gum line are harder, darker and bind very tightly on the root surfaces.

The removal of tartar established deeper down the roots of teeth is a far more tedious process. The formation of tartar is virtually painless, but the problem is that it has no inhibitions to form all the way down the entire length of the roots gradually displacing all the natural structures which attached to it. A tooth lost to gum disease often have their roots covered entirely in tartar.

This is how adult teeth shed.

Toothbrushing.

As dental plaque takes over a day to fully mature, it is in theory quite adequate to brush and floss the teeth once a day, or once every other day to prevent it accumulating to the point of causing harm. However, in reality, few people can clean their teeth so well at one time that all the plaque is removed and therefore more frequent brushing is recommended. It is important to use a brush which is in good condition. A worn and flared out toothbrush loses its brushing efficiency and becomes inefficient to remove debris from the gum line, which is a key objective. In an attempt to achieve this with a worn toothbrush, one may tend to use the central filaments of the brush with heavy strokes which will accelerate wear of the teeth. Eventually this will wear the enamel thin and expose the dentine underneath which is very sensitive. The gums will begin to recede and the roots of the teeth also begin to show. This is a very common and easy to do mistake, but gum recession with too much of the root showing is very difficult to repair. A smile which displays receded gums and bare tooth roots can be very unsightly. Make it a habit to change toothbrushes regularly.

Celebrities are very fond of wearing their teeth down with heavy brushing to make them look clean, but they also recede their gum lines in the process. The problem with enamel is that it cannot feel pain, and one can never be aware of it wearing thin.

Sensitivity and pain only occurs at dentine, and once dentine is reached, the wear is alarmingly faster because dentine is much softer. Abrasion caused by toothbrushing results in very deep and sensitive "abrasion cavities" and can be restored with composite resin fillings. In cases of extreme wear, porcelain veneers may be used to restore the whole surfaces of front teeth.

Toothbrushing is simply intended for the removal of soft dental plaque but never for the removal of heavy stains nor tartar. Heavy brushing will never make teeth look any whiter, but much yellower because the yellowness of dentine becomes more apparent.

How To Brush.

There are no hard and fast rules to toothbrushing, except for simple guidelines. The idea is to be able to cover as many areas of all your teeth, every surface from the top to the gum line without exerting too much pressure on any particular area on a tooth. It is important to strike a balance between removing the soft dental plaque yet at the same time cause minimal wear to the enamel. Repeats of heavy frictional forces focused on any one part the tooth surfaces would result in increased wear in the long term, and worn tooth structures don't grow back. Circular motions are better than heavy across-only motions, and do not concentrate only on the front teeth! Try and extend the brush filaments between your teeth, with up and down movements, getting the bristles to extend between them. Front, back, tops and gum lines are all gently brushed, including the far back surfaces of the last standing molar teeth. If you have kept your wisdom teeth, extra efforts are needed to brush at them. The head of the brush should be angled so that the filaments are at 45 degrees to the long axis of the tooth and should be placed at the gum line to allow the filaments to sweep at it gently. A back and forth light movement should be used.

Start at one side of the mouth and firstly brush the outside of your upper and lower teeth, going from one side of the mouth to another; do the same for the inside; and do the same for all of the chewing surfaces.

Choose a toothbrush with either soft or medium bristles, and the simpler the better, small and neat, straight and slim. However whatever you choose is fine so long as you feel comfortable with it, but change it when it feels worn. About every 1-2 months.

Hard brushes may scrub teeth very efficiently but are potentially more abrasive to teeth, wearing them faster in the long term.

Flossing.

As tooth brushes are unable to remove dental plaque in between the teeth, dental floss is used. It is passed between the teeth and used like a small "piece of cloth" to wipe clean those surfaces, clearing them of the dental plaque, which is quite soft. This technique is hard to teach, manipulating the floss is rather like learning how to use the "Chinese Chopsticks", but your dentist or hygienist will be more than happy to give you a good tuition after each regular check-up. Choosing the waxed or unwaxed types of floss is a personal choice. In addition, there is the "Superfloss" which is thicker, and has a hardened end for threading it through underneath dental bridges.

How To Floss.

Cut off a length of floss, 12 to 15 inches, twist it around the middle or index finger of both your hands, and guide it down between the teeth. Wipe the side surfaces of each tooth, up and down, to remove the dental plaque on these surfaces. Do not smack the floss down hard as it may hurt your gums. Do it gently, sliding it down between the teeth. If the floss catches on something, and shears to shreds, then you may have a rough filling. It will need to be checked by your dentist. Never use the floss with a sawing action because it will cut your gums. If the gums are healthy, there should never be any bleeding. Gum bleeding only indicates that you have an infection. Flossing is important and if you don't floss, you are simply leaving teeth uncleaned between them. You stand to lose your teeth because problems always occur in hidden areas; the in-between areas. Think about it, how often do you see a cavity right in the center of your front tooth? It never happens because the fronts of teeth are easily brushed! On the other hand, how many fillings are there between your back (or front) teeth? Commonly there's quite a few. These hidden areas are inaccessible to brushing and are considered to be stagnation areas.

INTERDENTAL BRUSHES.

These tiny brushes are very useful for removing plaque in between teeth, if spaces are large enough to allow them passing through. They are often used to clean underneath Dental Bridges. They are also useful to clean the wisdom teeth areas, or the back surfaces of the "last standing backtooth". They can reach the areas which the normal toothbrush is unable to clean.

ELECTRIC TOOTHBRUSHES.

The use of rotating electric toothbrushes for self-performed plaque control alone was shown to be nearly as equally effective as a more comprehensive set of oral hygiene devices, such as: toothbrush, floss, toothpick, interdental brush, etc. , in the hands of an ordinary person. Electric toothbrushes are really worth considering, but don't rely on them entirely and omit dental flossing.

If you are very heavy-handed and tend to brush your teeth across and very hard, you may consider using an electric toothbrush.

TOOTHPASTES.

Toothpastes offer little additional advantage to good mechanical toothbrushing in the removal of dental plaque, however its main advantage is that they contain fluoride, which helps to reduce decay. Their fresh flavours may add attractiveness to toothbrushing, encouraging it, and nowadays, chemicals are added for the whitening of teeth. However their concentrations are low and would require persistent usage in order to achieve satisfactory whitening effects. Try not to swallow toothpastes because the fluoride could make you feel sick, and only a tiny pea-sized amount is adequate.

MOUTHWASHES

Mouthwashes also offers additional advantage to good toothbrushing as it is virtually impossible to mechanically remove all the plaque in the mouth. They are also helpful when you have gum bleeding and mouthwashes can kill some bacteria in areas the brush cannot. Antibacterial mouthwashes can be used frequently without causing harm, and they are effective. Mouthwashes containing chlorhexidine gluconate are also good, and can often help to provide a temporary relief for soreness from mouth infections. They also help to discourage the formation of plaque on your teeth which is great, but the downside is that they can stain the teeth faster than your red wine, albeit harmless, chlorhexidine should be restricted to the odd occasion when you have serious gum bleedings, after a tooth extraction or a gum surgery. Mouthwashes however cannot penetrate far enough into deep gum pockets to control gum disease, and their penetration remains limited. Mouthwashes kills some of the bacteria, but not all.

23. Regular Care

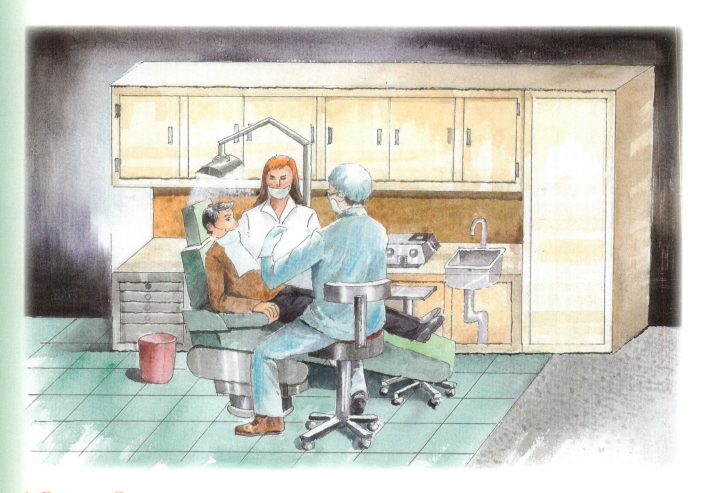

1. Regular Check-ups

Assuming that you now have good teeth, then you must maintain their conditions. It is important to have your teeth checked regularly to keep track of things, and allow any new problems which crept-in to be detected early and corrected. Once or twice a year is generally sufficient. New cavities are intercepted early with small fillings, and old crowns and fillings which have overhangs, are crumbling or are beginning to leak are quickly replaced. Ill-fitting dentures must be replaced because they can cause serious damage to the remaining teeth. If your dentures don't fit well in the mouth, not only can you not eat properly, but you stand to lose the rest of your teeth sooner. Root-filled teeth are checked for any recurrences of infections inside which can leak via the tips of their roots to form abscesses in the bone. These are all shown up on x-rays. Early re-root-treatment could save the tooth. Gum pockets are measured and x-rays could also be used to check for gums deteriorating because the low levels of bone around teeth would be clearly shown. Other various problems which were treated in previous visits are also re-checked. It is best that you stay with the same dentist because only he is most familiar with all of your past problems. General aspects in relation to your oral health are also checked, for example; mouth ulcers, signs of oral cancer, the health of your tongue, your palate and so on. Signs of general ill-health which commonly show up in the mouth are also looked for. For example, a red and sore tongue may be a sign of iron-deficiency anaemia.

2. Regular Cleaning - A Scale & Polish

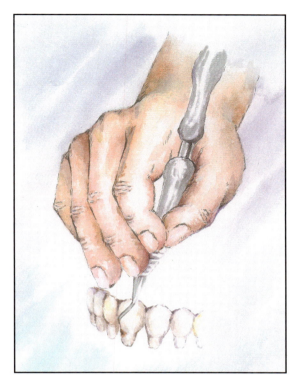

    Without regular cleaning, your only weapon against gum disease is your own toothbrush, and that alone is in the long term, grossly inadequate. It is important to realize that the slow progression of gum disease is caused by the slow and gradual build-up of tartar forming down the tooth roots below the gums which is never obvious to the naked eye and is not removable by your toothbrush. The tartar formed in 3 months can become so hard and so tightly bonded to your roots that you will need a kitchen fork to scrape it off by yourself, even if you know what you are doing. Even dentists seek their colleagues for help.

    The irreversible processes of detachment of the gums and the alarming disappearance of bone from the tooth roots is so gradual that it is totally painless from start to finish. We call this process "slowly but surely". Gum bleeding may be a first sign of gum disease, but it only relates to the very superficial infection of the gums and its absence does not rule out deeper destruction. In the fortunate event that pus does get trapped, the pressure build-up causes painful gum abscess which reveal the problem, but if the pus is successful in spilling itself out continuously into the mouth, the process remains unsuspected as there is never any pain. Smokers are at particular risk as tobacco stains and tartar form much more rapidly and abundantly to cause significant deterioration of the gums. Heavy smokers may need extra cleaning sessions each year for this reason. Regular cleaning, at least once a year, is absolutely needed for the long term health of your gums, and it should always be a lifetime discipline and not the "one-off effort". It is good practice to have a highest level of personal and oral hygiene. Preventing gum disease does demand a lifelong commitment. Never tolerate the tartar and stains on your teeth to remain for too long. They can house millions of harmful bacteria, and bear in mind, if you do have pus in the mouth, you're likely to be sharing this too with your spouse!

A Word About Pregnancy.

During pregnancy, regular check-ups remain important but it is best to avoid x-rays completely as far as possible. If there should be any need for a root-canal treatment, the tooth is treated and dressed temporarily with the aim to stabilize the condition, but is completed only after the baby is born. Other minimally invasive treatments such as routine cleaning, fillings and crowns are quite safe to do during pregnancy. Due to the hormonal changes in the body during this period, the gums are less capable to defend against the normal levels of bacteria in the mouth, leading to "pregnancy gingivitis." The best way to counterbalance this is simply to step-up your oral hygiene, in the most meticulous fashion. If there is no dental plaque on the gums for most of the time, you will have mostly "no problems". Dairy products such as milk and cheese will provide you with calcium, vitamin A and D which is needed for the normal development of the baby teeth. Fish is a good source of vitamin A and plenty of sunshine will help the skin to form vitamin D which is essential for the absorption of calcium. Try to avoid taking any medicines during pregnancy as far as possible, especially the tetracycline group of antibiotics, and avoid aspirin altogether.

N. B. Aspirin (acetyl salicylate) is never given to a child under the age of 12yrs. old as it has potential to cause a neurological condition known as Reye's Syndrome. Aspirin (at 300mg dosage) remains to be a very effective anti-inflammatory pain-killer for adults. However it does interfere with the blood clotting as it prevents the aggregation of the platelets on the wound which forms the very first step of the clotting process. This is why aspirin is never prescribed to patients who have just had a tooth extracted. On the other hand, because of this particular feature of aspirin, it is commonly used as a blood thinner for people who have high blood pressure or heart problems.

24. Dental Phobia !

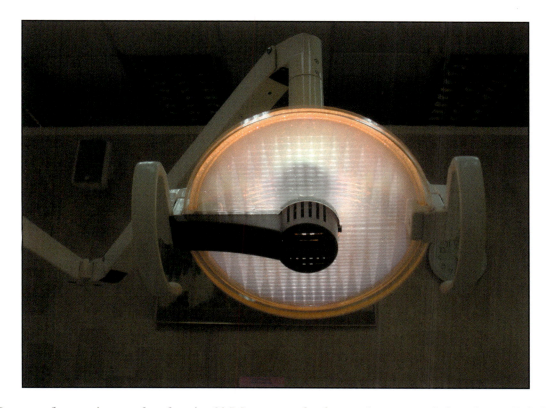

Do you fear going to the dentist ?! Most people do, and you won't be alone. It is by far the commonest reason for people to avoid getting their teeth fixed, desperate as they are, but they just cannot bring themselves to even make an appointment.

They know that their teeth are all in dreadful states and it may have affected their social lives and personalities. They don't like talking too much and won't smile readily. They're even too embarrassed to show them to a dentist because of their conditions.

In this ultra-modern, high-tech age of dentistry, the problem of dental phobia still exists, and it affects a large proportion of the population. Despite the fact that good dental appearance is becoming increasingly important in today's affluent and health-oriented society, dental phobia or related anxieties still exists amongst many. Technological advances in dentistry which have provided great sophistication to the profession have not been able to quash the fears within the anxious patient.

Whenever the topic is mentioned, the first thing on the mind is the sound of the drill, sitting on the dental chair having a light shining on the face, and getting an injection in the mouth. Most people are afraid of needles in the mouth, and particularly children. The sight of the needle could literally send a child leaping right out of the chair, climb out through the window, and disappear off into the fields. It really does happen! Some people are afraid of the volumes of water in the mouth and they find it difficult not to swallow more than half of it. Some people simply dread the numb feeling in the mouth afterwards. The vibrations in the head are never pleasant but despite all of this, it never actually turns out to be all as painful as they had feared!! It's mostly a psychological phenomena, and the fear within is mostly based on a highly exaggerated version of the reality.

Culture also reinforces this fear and it's human nature to joke about these stressful experiences. The association of dental treatments with extreme pain often stems from bad childhood experiences. Whilst dental treatment maybe unpleasant at most, and the thoughts of it brings shivers down your spine, what's probably the most painful memory of it all was the throbbing toothache itself, and the anxious worries of having a tooth which was already excruciatingly painful, drilled ! How could it possibly not be painful ?!

An anxious child with a huge and painful cavity is virtually trapped between the devil and the deep blue sea. Fear and anxiety always mounts once seated on the dental chair; they'd grasp at the armrests and tense-up all over. Their hearts pound so quickly you could almost see it in their mouths. To their astonishment, the very minute after an injection was given, the pain disappears! It was like an anti-climax.

Dentistry today is in fact remarkably painless thanks to the wonder of anaesthetics. In the historic days, teeth were forcefully pulled out of their sockets without anaesthetics and imaginary visions of these clouded the dental profession. Today, once the tooth is numbed, the rest is easy and over in minutes!! The anaesthetics also constrict the blood vessels and so there is actually very little bleeding except for a drop on the handkerchief. (Without anaesthetics, the bleeding would be very profuse).

By the time the anaesthetics wear off the solid clot had already formed and this clot left neatly in place plugs the socket.

Dental phobia is very common, and some people would rather let their gums and teeth deteriorate to their very ends and would rather endure all the pain at home than to seek for an appointment. It's actually more painful that way. Sleeping it off was their motto.

PREVENTION. -WHAT YOU CAN DO FOR YOURSELF.

What you can do is to prevent the cavities by yourself by maintaining the highest level of oral hygiene as possible. The cause of tooth decay and gum disease is identified to be bacterial plaque, and poor oral hygiene is always responsible for these. Children are more prone to decay mostly because they never really brush so well. Sweets could never do any harm without plaque. Some people gag easily with toothbrushes in their mouths and so choosing a tiny toothbrush, or a baby brush may be useful for the more sensitive areas. If you have already a lot of fillings, crowns and bridges in the mouth, and had a lot of cavities as a child, you might benefit from using a daily gargle of fluoride mouthrinses which are available at your local chemist. Additionally you can ask your dentist to give you a fluoride gel treatment once a year. One fluoride gel treatment takes only 3 minutes. After every meal, always rinse your mouth with water, or you might drink a small glass of plain water just before you leave the table. Chewing xylitol gum is quite useful because it stimulates your flow of saliva which washes away your sweet meal and neutralizes the acids.

PREVENTIVE DENTISTRY. -WHAT THE PROFESSION CAN DO FOR YOU.

There are prevention treatments which are intended to prevent the needs for those drills and fills, pulling and replacing teeth and they are by far the most important yet painless ones. They're about starting children at their early ages for regular check-ups, regular cleaning and polishing teeth, topical fluoride application and fissure sealants to prevent decay, teaching them comprehensively how to brush their teeth, and providing braces to straighten their teeth. Most of these are relatively painless and if they should cause dental phobia, they couldn't truly be justified. Prevention starts with children. They must never be allowed to suffer the needs for dreadful treatments if at all possible, otherwise these could trigger their dental phobia. The main prevention treatment for adults is the regular checking and cleaning every six months, for life.

How To Deal With It When You Have Tooth Problems.

1. Find yourself a dentist who is caring and is willing to spend time for you. Dentists who are very busy would be less able to attend to your anxious conditions and it's best to find one who will spare extra time for you. Many dental offices nowadays have audio-visual equipment which can help to calm your nerves down. Some even have personal headphones for you to wear during the procedure. You can bring in your favourite music, or even your favourite music videos.

2. If you fear the pain of mouth injections, anaesthetic gels can firstly be applied to the gums 3 minutes prior to the injection. This way you won't feel a thing. If you fear the water going down your throat, you may request for use of a rubber dam which isolates the tooth to be treated from the rest of your mouth.

3. Sedation methods are also available if you are indeed very anxious.
Many dental offices have "laughing gas" or nitrous oxide mixed with oxygen, and it is delivered via a small mask.
Anaesthetists are also available nowadays in private dental offices and arrangements can be made for their services. A light sedation can be conducted during the treatment procedure. It's best to start with a first check-up just to realize the extents of your problems and to discuss the treatment plan, the number of visits that are necessary and the costs involved. Ideally if an anaesthetist is to assist in your treatments, most or all of your major problems are tackled together in the single session. Children can benefit from this service.

4. Choose the highest grade of materials available for restoring your back teeth; cast fillings in gold or ceramics are likely to serve you well longer than amalgams. Amalgams are intended for replacements over time as they tend to deteriorate, distort, or disintegrate. Gold fillings, on the other hand have better potential to last for decades in your mouth without disintegrating. Porcelain fillings are beautiful and could remain undistorted, but they could fracture with heavy biting.

5. Maintain the highest level of oral hygiene you know how, and keep up your regular check-ups and dental cleanings.
Never use a worn toothbrush because it can do more harm than good, change a new one often, and never beyond 3 months.
Flossing your teeth is as important as brushing them, i. e. you musn't leave the in-betweens of your teeth unattended.

6. Maintain a balanced diet, never to be deficient in calcium or vitamin C, eat plenty of fruits and drink plenty of water.
Calcium is needed to maintain the bone healthy around your teeth, and vitamin C is needed for collagen synthesis which makes up your gum tissues and the collagen fibres which attach the teeth to the bone.

7. Do not smoke because it encourages more rapid formation of tartar and stains in your mouth which causes deterioration of your gums.

8. Avoid brushing your teeth too hard or the bristles will destructively wear away the enamel, exposing the sensitive dentine.
   Avoid prolonged sucking of grapefruit, lemons or citrus fruits because their acids can erode your teeth, dissolving them to their pulps. If you tend to grind your teeth at night, you must wear a nightguard during sleeping.

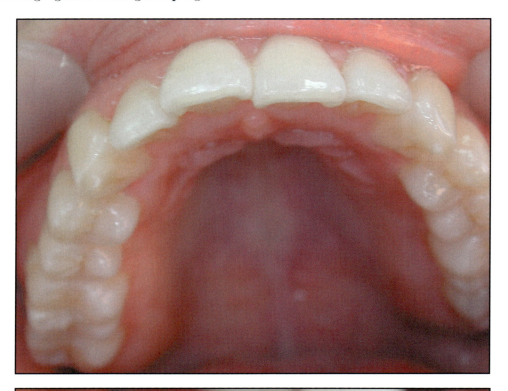

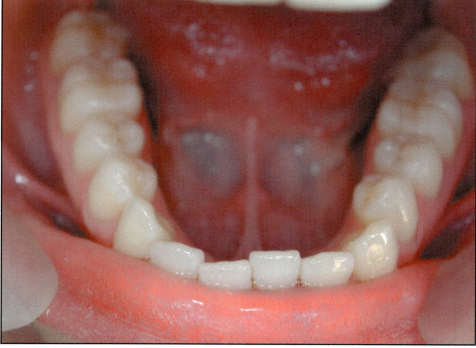

If you can keep your teeth as clean as this, you'll have absolutely nothing to worry about at each dental check-up!

25. A List Of 20 Precautions.

1. Brush your teeth for 3 minutes each time, twice a day using a soft or medium brush and a pea-size of fluoride toothpaste and always floss them afterwards. Do this in the morning <u>before</u> breakfast, and at night <u>just before</u> bedtime.
2. Never use the same toothbrush for over 3 months, and certainly not for 6 months. Change your toothbrush regularly, every 2 months is best, and the same goes for the replaceable brushes for electric toothbrushes. A good habit is to buy a few in a multi-pack each time so that new brushes are always available. Choose either soft or medium bristles.
3. If you have dental bridges in the mouth, make an effort to clean underneath them with inter-dental brushes.
4. If you have wisdom teeth in the mouth, make cleaning at them a top priority. Using a baby toothbrush just for them is ideal.
   If your teeth are crooked, or have many fillings in the mouth, make more efforts to brush and floss at them, as a top priority.
5. **ABRASION**-Do not brush heavily across at your teeth as this would rapidly wear the enamel, recede the gums, and expose the sensitive dentine at the necks of the teeth. This sensitivity is discomforting and commonly confused with tooth decay.
6. **ATTRITION**-Do not grind your teeth. This will rapidly wear the biting surfaces and shorten all the teeth simultaneously.
   Wear a night guard during sleeping if you tend to grind your teeth at night.
7. **EROSION**-Do not suck on lemons, grapefruits or oranges for prolonged periods of time everyday as this habit will eventually erode all your front teeth and you will then need a mouthful of crowns.
8. Do not use your teeth to bite on bottle-caps, chew pencils, chew bones, or crack open seafoods such as crab or lobster shells.
   If you have front teeth porcelain veneers or crowns, avoid nibbling on nuts and seeds.
9. Avoid too many sugary snacks between meals, and especially never just before you go to sleep. Avoid sticky sweets.
10. Have a rinse of water just after a sweet meal, and if you eat out at a restaurant, have a last sip of water just before you leave.
11. Always wear a mouth guard during all contact sports.
12. If your upper front teeth are very forward protruding, ask your orthodontist to correct them before they are knocked one day.
13. Have your teeth checked and cleaned once or twice a year, and if you are a heavy smoker, have them cleaned 3 times a year.
14. If you are a heavy smoker, don't touch alcohol. The two combined work synergistically over decades to cause oral cancer.
15. If food always trap between teeth after every meal, have it checked to see if there are rough crowns or fillings which need to be corrected. Trapping food between teeth everyday, over time, will lead to toothaches and tooth losses.
16. If you have dentures for your back teeth, wear them everyday to prevent the remaining

teeth from drifting. If you leave your dentures out for too long, the teeth would drift and they may never fit again. Do not wear dentures during sleeping.

17. If you have Dental Implants in the mouth, keep them as clean as you can. Never grind on Dental Implant supported teeth.
18. Drink plenty of water during the day to keep the mouth moist, especially if you have to take a lot of daily medicines.
19. Have a balanced diet. Iron deficiency anaemia can result in more mouth ulcers, and this can also occur with deficiencies of vitamin B. Keep an eye also on your daily calcium intake. Simply ensure that you are indeed, not deficient in calcium.

    A glass of non-fat milk each day will provide you with almost one-third of your daily calcium needs. Dairy products such as cheese and yogurt are also good sources. Excess intake of alcohol and coffee, or stress, will reduce calcium absorption.
20. Chewing xylitol gum, apples, celery and carrots after a meal is always preferable to the very sweet desert offerings.

Further Reading.

1. The Art and Science of Operative Dentistry-Sturdevant, Roberson, Heymann, Swift.
2. An Outline of Periodontics- J.D. Manson.
3. Journal of Clinical Periodontology, supplement 5, volume 30- Jan Lindhe.
4. Oral Implantology-Schroeder, Sutter, Buser, Krekeler.
5. Contemporary Orthodontics- Profitt.
6. Traumatic Dental Injuries- J.O. Andreasen, F.M. Andreasen, L.K. Bakland, M.T. Flores.
7. Contemporary Oral and Maxillofacial Surgery- Peterson, Ellis, Hupp, Tucker.
8. Contemporary Fixed Prosthodontics- Rosenstiel, Land, Fujimoto.
9. Introduction to Dental Materials- Richard Van Noort.
10. Applied Dental Materials- John F. McCabe.

INDEX

A
abscess	20,52
abrasion	46
amalgam	36
anaemia	104
anatomy	1
antibacterial mouthwashes	103
antibiotics	51
appearance zone	72
aspirin	106
attrition	45

B
bacteraemia	52
bad breath	92
bleaching	81
bottle feeding	12
bridge	64
braces	24
brushing	12,101
bruxism	45

C
calcium	96
cast fillings	37
calculus	101
canine	1
ceramic	40
composite resin(bonding)	35
cosmetic dentistry	70
crossbite	77
crowding(overcrowding)	24
crowns(caps)	41

D
decay(dental caries)	30
dental implants	66
dental phobia	107
dental trauma	55
dentine	3
dentures	62
diabetes	100
dry mouth(xerostomia)	92

E
enamel	3
electric toothbrushes	103
erosion	46
evolution	24
extra space	25
extrinsic staining	80

F
facebow	28
fillings	35
fissure sealants	16,33,60
flossing	102
food for teeth	94
functions of teeth	5,6,7,8
fluoride	15,31,32

G
gingivitis	20
gingivectomy	22
grinding	45
gum disease	19
gum line	97

H
halitosis	92
headgear	28
heart valve infections	52

I
incisor	1
infections	52
immediate dental implant	61
impacted	48
inlays	37
intrinsic staining	81

J
jaw correction	74
jawjoint	7,56,88

L
laminates	83,84
lingual brackets	78

M
mal-occlusion	87
materials	39
mercury	36
metals	39
minerals	95
molars	2
mouthguards	56
mouthwashes	103

N
nerve	3,16,43
nightguards	45
nutrition	95

O
occlusion	87
orthodontics	24
oral cancer	54
overbite	76
overhangs	58,104
overjet	76

P
plaque	100
periodontal disease	19
periodontitis	20
premolars	2,25
pregnancy	106
prevention	10,108

Q
quality of life	5

R
regular check-ups	104
regular cleaning	105
retainers	28
root canal treatment	43
root decay	92
root planing	25
rubber dam	82

S
scaling	21
sensitivity	46,101
sinusitis	53
smoking	20

T
tartar	101
teething	11
toothpastes	103

V
veneers	83

W
wisdom teeth	16,48,52

X
x-rays	104
xylitol	31,112

Y
yellow teeth	79,81

LaVergne, TN USA
21 August 2009
155524LV00003B